Dedications, Second Edition

For the grands: Kathryn Hope and Aaron James.

Jan Ledford

To the many technicians and assistants who have allowed me to be useful in their training.

Val Sanders

Dedications, First Edition

For my part, I would like to dedicate this work to some special teachers who whet my curiosity for scientific things: Beatrice Harris (who taught me the scientific method), George M. Hood (who showed me the rings around Saturn via telescope), Linda Bennett (who introduced me to the microscopic world of the paramecium), Robert Sipe (who let me use class time to work on a science project that made it to state competition), Carole Calvert Vann (who made botany and ecology incredibly interesting), and Sally Blackwell (who let me grow nearly a hundred green bean plants in her classroom).

Jan Ledford

I would like to dedicate my portion of this endeavor to my family: to my husband, Chuck, whose unending support could never be matched; to my children, Riley, Zachary, and Carlye, who have taught me what is important in life; and to my parents, John and Juanita Nordin, who encouraged me to pursue my goals.

Val Sanders

D1354835

Contents

Dedications...*iii*

Acknowledgments...*viii*

About the Authors ....*ix*

The Study Icons...*xi*

Chapter 1. The Slit Lamp 1

Chapter 2. The Basic Slit Lamp Exam..11

Chapter 3. A Magnified Tour of the Normal Eye..........................33

Chapter 4. Illumination Techniques...45

Chapter 5. Slit Lamp Findings 57

Chapter 6. The Problematic Examination 85

Chapter 7. The Postoperative Eye 103

Chapter 8. History Mystery 117

Chapter 9. Contact Lens Evaluation for Nonfitters.....................123

References..*135*

Index..*139*

Acknowledgments

We would like to gratefully acknowledge the kind help of so many wonderful people. First, we appreciate the editorial advice given by Bob Campbell, MD; Ken Daniels, OD; and Jeff Freund, COMT. Dori Witten and Pete Leadman, of Topcon, assisted by providing photographs of Topcon slit lamps as well as the user's manuals. We acknowledge the use of certain photographs from books in SLACK's original Ophthalmic Technical Skills Series. Collin Ledford was a willing photographic model, as were Susan Dumont, Riley and Zachary Sanders, Karen Brown, Tammy Langley, and John Nordin. We also thank those providers and technical staff at Eyesight Associates of Middle Georgia who referred appropriate patients for photography: David Grogan, PA-C; Matt Dixon, OD; Louis Schlesinger, OD; and Monte Murphy, OD. Others who assisted in photograph and illustration procurement are Patrick Caroline, COT, FCLSA; Jane Beeman, COA, FCLSA (of Bausch & Lomb/Polymer Technology); Tim Koch, FCLSA; Sheila Nemeth, COMT; and J. Michael Coppinger, MA, CRA. Denise Cunningham, COA, COPRA, had the idea for the illumination mnemonic, although we later developed our own. Jim Ledford, PA-C; Charles Shaller, MD; and Johnny Gayton, MD graciously loaned us reference materials. ILAMO (International Library, Archives, and Museum of Optometry); Joseph T. Barr, OD; and Marcia Meyer (FDA) helped find references, as well. We are indebted to the following people, who provided technical advice: Tammy Langley, COT; Todd Hostetter, COMT; Ken Woodworth, COMT; Donna Knight, COT, CRA; Susan Clark-Rath, SA; and Michael Novak, MD. Finally, we appreciate the good folks at SLACK Incorporated who have provided us with a way to share our knowledge with our colleagues.

About the Authors

Those engaged in the happy profession of ophthalmic medical assisting are beginning to know Jan Ledford, COMT, as a premier writer of training material and texts. *The Slit Lamp Primer, Second Edition* is her fouteenth book for ophthalmic medical personnel (OMP), but she is probably best known for her first two review books: *Certified Ophthalmic Assistant Exam Review Manual* and *Certified Ophthalmic Technician Exam Review Manual*. She is also the co-author of *The Crystal Clear Guide to Sight For Life*, a lay-oriented book on all things ocular for people over 40.

In 1995, Jan was selected as the Series Editor of *The Basic Bookshelf for Eyecare Professionals*. She admits that she has a soft spot in her heart for OMP who are working their way through the ranks. "When I started in the field back in 1982, there was basically one published text for ophthalmic assistants," she notes. "In *The Basic Bookshelf*, we have been able to go way beyond anything that's been done before. The Series is full of grass-roots stuff; things you can use in the exam room and on certification exams. I wish this material had been available when I first started."

Jan makes her home in Franklin, NC with her husband Jim (a Physician's Assistant, PhD, and medical examiner) and son Collin. They have four cats, which she insists on at least mentioning since pictures are not allowed.

Val Sanders started her career in ophthalmology in 1979 as a tech (given 2 weeks' "training") for three doctors in Seattle, Wash. She read everything she could find in order to perfect her technical skills. The doctors she worked with believed that her advancement would benefit the practice, so they answered her innumerable questions and encouraged her to take continuing education programs, when available. In 1982, she took and passed the certification exam for ophthalmic technician. Two years later, she relocated to Georgia and joined a solo practice. She was soon promoted to clinical supervisor and played a part in the training of dozens of ophthalmic medical personnel as the practice grew.

In 1992, Val completed the certification as a retinal angiographer. Today, Val works as an administrator for a busy ophthalmology practice but still ventures into the lanes to stay in touch with the medical side of things. She assists in preparing presentations for staff, patients, and the ophthalmic community. In her off time, she can be found at home with the kids or working on the house.

The Study Icons

The Basic Bookshelf for Eyecare Professionals is quality educational material designed for professionals in all braches of eyecare. Because so many of you want to expand your careers, we have made a special effort to include information needed for certification exams. When these study icons appear in the margin of a *Series* book, it is your cue that the material next to the icon is listed as a criteria item for a certification examination. Please use this key to identify the appropriate icon:

OptP	paraoptometric
OptA	paraoptometric assistant
OptT	paraoptometric technician
OphA	ophthalmic assistant
OphT	ophthalmic technician
OphMT	ophthalmic medical technologist[*]
Srg	ophthalmic surgical assisting subspecialty
CL	contact lens registry
Optn	opticianry
RA	retinal angiographer

*Note: Because this icon applies to the entire book, it will not appear anywhere on the pages.

Chapter 1

The Slit Lamp

KEY POINTS

- The slit lamp microscope is uniquely designed to give a three-dimensional view of the eye and its structures.

- Because the slit lamp provides a binocular view, the location of abnormalities can be determined with great precision.

- The magnification of the microscope is provided by the oculars and the objective lenses.

- The slit lamp should be located in a room free of dust and excessive heat or humidity.

- A supply of bulbs, fuses, and chin papers should be kept on hand.

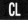

Instrumentation

The eye is one of the most fascinating structures of the body. A great deal of this fascination hinges on the fact that it is the only organ that we can look directly into without having to cut and/or insert a special scope.

The slit lamp is a microscope designed specifically to examine the eye. It is composed of a microscope and a light source. The microscope is binocular; that is, it has two eyepieces, giving the binocular observer a stereoscopic (3-dimensional) view of the eye. Thus, another name for the instrument is the biomicroscope. Because the ocular structures can be examined dimensionally, the location of abnormalities can be determined with great precision.

The slit lamp is used to examine the external ocular adnexa, external eye, anterior chamber, iris, and crystalline lens. The anterior face of the vitreous may also be visible if the lens is clear.

Although there are numerous manufacturers and models of slit lamps, there are basically only two styles. The first utilizes a horizontal prism reflected light source (Figure 1-1). The second has a vertical illumination source (Figure 1-2).

The microscope is mounted on a stage that is designed for movement of the microscope and positioning of the patient. Microscope position is controlled by a joystick. Moving in and out (toward and away from the patient) allows the observer to focus the microscope at various depths. Twisting the joystick (or a wheel at its base) moves the microscope up and down, allowing the examiner to view various structures. The joystick can also be used to move the microscope from side to side, allowing scanning and easy movement from one eye to the other.

The microscope has various magnification settings. Most instruments have magnification abilities ranging from 6X to 40X. Magnification power is changed by flipping a lever or turning a dial (Figures 1-3A and 1-3B). (The power of the oculars is fixed. You are actually changing the objective lens when you change magnification). This can be done during the exam itself and does not interrupt the observer or the patient. Magnifications of 6X, 10X, and 16X are adequate for most exam purposes. Higher magnifications can be achieved by removing the standard oculars and inserting stronger-powered ones.

The actual magnification of what you see through the slit lamp is derived by multiplying the power of the oculars with the power of the objective lens. Thus, if your oculars are 10X and the objective lens is 1.6X, the total magnification will be 16X.

In addition to magnification, some oculars have an internal line or grid for measuring ocular structures. Other eyepieces incorporate an angle scale that is very useful in fitting and evaluating toric contact lenses. An ocular with a cross hair reticule is used in slit lamp photography.

The light source of the slit lamp is unique to this microscope and is the feature that makes it so adaptable for looking at the eye. The light is controlled by a transformer, which provides various voltage settings. The beam of light can be changed in intensity, height, width, direction or angle, and color during the exam with the flick of a lever or turn of a dial (Figure 1-4A and 1-4B). The majority of the microscopic eye exam is done with the light beam set at maximum height but with a narrow width that produces a slit of light, hence the name slit lamp. In addition, the light source (illuminator) moves independently of the microscope unit, making various types of illumination and views of ocular structures possible. A click-stop indicates when the light is directly aligned with the microscope. However, most illumination techniques require that the light be positioned at an angle to the scope. A marked dial (angle scale index) at the base of the arm indicates degrees (Figure 1-5). The microscope

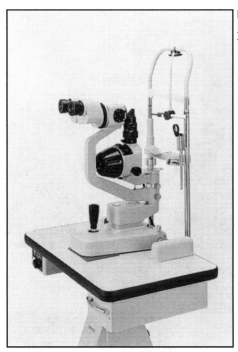

Figure 1-1. Topcon slit lamp model SL-2E with horizontal prism reflected light source. (Photo courtesy Topcon.)

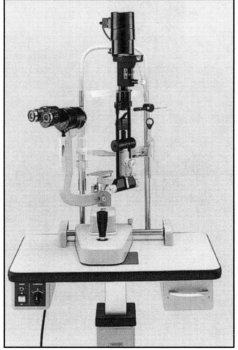

Figure 1-2. Topcon slit lamp model SL-3E with vertical illumination source. (Photo courtesy Topcon.)

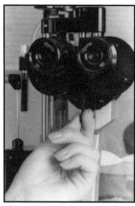

Figure 1-3A. Magnification may be changed by flipping a lever... (Photo by Mark Arrigoni.)

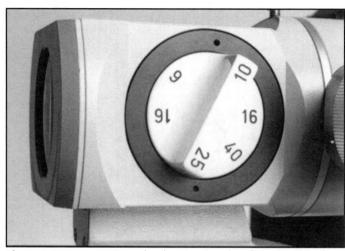

Figure 1-3B...or rotating a knob. (Reprinted with permission from *Ophthalmic Photography*, SLACK Incorporated.)

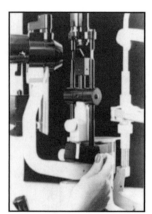

Figure 1-4A. The light beam is controlled by knobs... (Photo by Mark Arrigoni.)

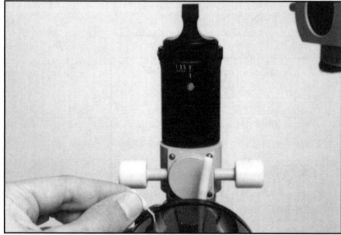

Figure 1-4B. ...or levers (Reprinted with permission from *Ophthalmic Photography*, SLACK Incorporated. Photo by Steve Carlton.)

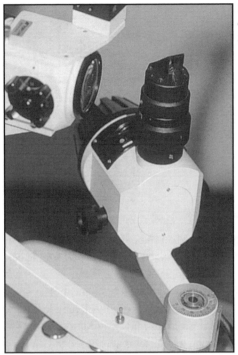

Figure 1-5. The angle of the light source is indicated by a dial at the base of the arm. (Photo by Val Sanders.)

and light are coordinated so that the structure to be viewed is magnified and illuminated. This can be altered by moving the slit image off center, as is required by some illumination techniques (discussed in Chapter 4).

While white light is used for most examinations, there are several colored filters that can be utilized, as well. The cobalt blue filter is used in conjunction with fluorescein dye. The dye pools in areas where the corneal epithelium is broken or absent. The blue light excites the fluorescein, which then takes on a yellowish glow.

The green filter obscures anything that is red (hence the pseudonym red-free light); thus, blood vessels or hemorrhages appear black. This increases contrast, revealing the path and pattern of inflamed blood vessels. Areas of the episclera where lymphocytes (infection-fighting white blood cells) have gathered in response to an inflammatory or immune response will appear as yellow spots under the red-free light. Fleischer ring (seen in keratoconus, see Chapter 5) can also be viewed satisfactorily with the red-free filter.

Some instruments also have a diffuser, which is a piece of frosted glass or plastic that flips in front of the illuminator. The diffuser scatters the light, causing an even spread of light over the entire ocular surface. The filters are placed by flipping a lever (Figure 1-6).

Patient positioning is achieved by an attached head rest unit that includes a moveable chin cup and a stationary forehead band. There may also be a strap that can be fastened behind the patient's head to ensure stability. Most models also include a moveable fixation light, which gives the patient a target to look at while his or her eye is being examined. There may also be grips for the patient to hold on to, mounted on the side of the head rest unit. (Patient positioning is discussed in Chapter 2.) Some units have a breath shield attached to the microscope arm for the convenience and comfort of both operator and patient.

Figure 1-6. Changing filters. (Photo by Mark Arrigoni.)

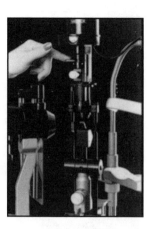

In addition to outright observation, the slit lamp is used when removing foreign bodies, epilating lashes, trimming sutures, fitting contact lenses, inserting punctal plugs, and performing certain minor surgery procedures (corneal scraping, anterior chamber tap, etc).

Other parts or functions of the eye may be examined with additional equipment. The angle structures of the eye can be examined with the slit lamp if a gonio lens is used. A Hruby lens, high power indirect lens, fundus contact lens, or a Goldmann 3-mirror lens may be used to view the vitreous, retina, and optic nerve with the slit lamp. The Goldmann tonometer is attached to the slit lamp and is commonly used to measure intraocular pressure (IOP). An observation tube can be affixed to allow a second person to view structures and procedures simultaneously with the examiner. Some models can be equipped with an attachment for noncontact specular microscopy. Other instruments that are often used in conjunction with the slit lamp are the A-scan ultrasound, the pachymeter, the laser, the potential acuity meter, the 35 mm camera, and the video camera. All of these techniques are beyond the purpose of this book, but most are described in other *Series* titles.

Instrument Maintenance

The slit lamp should be set up in a room that is free of dust. The first act of maintenance that should be performed daily is to cover an unused instrument. Excessive heat or humidity, as well as exposure to direct sunlight, should also be avoided.

When replacing the main illumination bulb, first turn off the instrument and disconnect the power source. In slit lamps with a vertical illumination source, the bulb is on the top of the illumination tower (Figure 1-7). In instruments with a horizontal prism, the bulb housing must be loosened by turning (Figure 1-8). If the bulb housing has a connecting plug and cable, wiggle gently to loosen it. (Never disconnect any plug by pulling on the cable.) Consult your user's manual for details. Make sure to be careful with the old bulb; it may be hot. Use a tissue or cloth to protect your fingers. It is also helpful to know what kind of bulb you are dealing with (ie, push-pull, lift-out key, bayonet mount, etc) before trying to remove the bulb. If a bulb is difficult to remove, wiggle it gently. Do not force the bulb; the jacket may break from the metal neck.

While the bulb is out of the instrument, check the metal contacts (Figure 1-7). These may be cleaned with a cotton tip moistened with isopropyl alcohol. If there is any corrosion, try removing it with a pencil eraser. If that does not work, try a knife or file. (Make sure the instrument is unplugged first.)

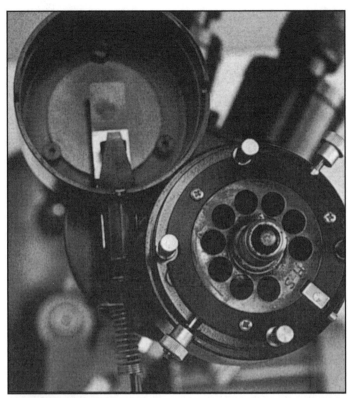

Figure 1-7. Bulb and lamp housing of a vertical illumination type slit lamp. There is oxidation on the contact in the cover.

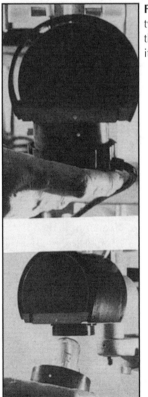

Figure 1-8. Bulb housing of a horizontal prism reflected light source type slit lamp. The white dots are aligned when removing or inserting the bulb assembly into the housing. The bulb housing is turned to lock it into place.

Figure 1-9. If the mirror cannot be cleaned with compressed air or camel's hair brush, a lens wipe can be used.

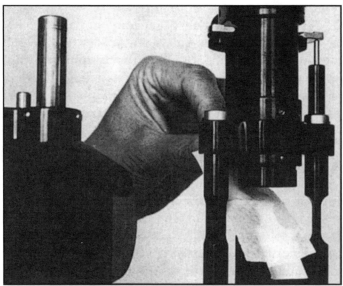

When handling the new bulb, also use a tissue, cloth, or bulb holder. Finger prints on the bulb can reduce illumination. Carefully reassemble the bulb housing. If the housing is not correctly seated, illumination may be uneven or partially obscured in some models.

The bulb for the fixation target will also need to be replaced periodically. The target itself is removed to expose the bulb, which is of the push-pull type.

Before replacing a fuse, disconnect the instrument. Some fuses must be loosened with a screwdriver. See the instructions for your microscope. Always replace a fuse with another of the proper AMP rating. This rating is engraved into the metal end of the fuse jacket. Taping an extra fuse directly to the instrument will save time, since maintenance always seems to be needed during high-traffic patient hours! Bulb life is extended if you operate the instrument at the lowest voltage setting. If you do use higher voltage, be sure to turn the setting back down to the lowest before turning the instrument on or off.

Many instrument models provide a supply of chin rest papers that can be changed between patients. The papers are held in place by pins or screws, which are easily removed to allow replacement.

Do not touch any lens or mirror with your finger or any hard object. Lenses and mirrors may be cleaned with compressed air or a cleaning brush. A lint-free cloth moistened with alcohol may possibly be used (Figure 1-9), but check with the manufacturer for recommendations. Alcohol may affect the glue of a mounted lens. Never spray any type of cleaner onto the instrument. If necessary, the mirror of the vertical illumination tower type of microscope may be removed. To do so, tilt the illumination column slightly (about 10 degrees) and gently pull the mirror out of its housing by grasping the tab at the top. If there is no tab, you can tease the mirror up by using a flat head optical screwdriver or the sharp end of a pencil to push it from the bottom. The mirror can then be cleaned under a gentle stream of cool water. Use a lint-free lens wipe or a cotton swab to pat the mirror dry; do not rub.

The glide plate needs to be clean in order for the instrument to move smoothly. Clean it with a dry cloth. If the ball bearing is dirty, it will leave dirty track marks on the plate. Wipe repeatedly with a dry cloth until no more tracks appear. If your user's manual does not warn against it, you might also clean the friction plate by wiping gently with a cloth moistened with alcohol. If you use alcohol, you should treat the plate with silicone or WD-40™ after every fifth cleaning. This helps negate the drying effects of the alcohol.

Plastic parts such as the chin rest and forehead rest may be cleaned with a mild neutral detergent and water. Other cleansers are not recommended. The forehead rest of some models is metal padded with rubber; the rubber will be ruined if alcohol is used to clean it. Clean up any spills (dye, tears, etc) as soon as they occur.

It is possible to adjust certain features of some slit lamp models. The slit width control of models such as the one in Figure 1-2 can be tightened if the slit beam tends to collapse. In this case, you should use a screwdriver to tighten the screw in the knob's center. The light source of these models is designed to incline. However, if the inclination mechanism becomes too loose, it may be tightened by turning the screws on the pivot. Consult your instruction manual before attempting any adjustments.

The base of the instrument should be moved to its back-most position and the stage locked after every examination. In addition, the instrument should be turned off when not in use.

Chapter 2

The Basic Slit Lamp Exam

KEY POINTS

- Patient education is an important aspect of the slit lamp exam.

- A comfortable patient is a more cooperative patient.

- Before beginning, adjust the ocular power and pupillary distance (PD).

- Using lower voltage settings preserves bulb life.

- Manipulate the microscope with one hand on the light source and the other hand on the joystick.

- Developing and following an examination protocol will help ensure quality patient care.

- Accurate, legible documentation is the last step of any slit lamp examination.

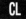

Patient Positioning

Before positioning the patient, check to make sure that the slit lamp stage is locked in the position farthest away from the head support unit. Also, fold the tonometer arm completely out of the way if it was left in position. If the stage is not locked, the microscope may roll forward and bash the headrest unit, jarring the delicate optics and light system. If the tonometer arm is in position when the stage is not locked, and the slit lamp then rolls forward, the tonometer could hit the patient in the face or eye. Safety first!

Explain the examination to the patient. The slit lamp may look formidable or frightening, especially to a child. Reassure the patient that this is just a fancy microscope.

Ask the patient to lean forward and place his or her chin in the chin rest and the forehead against the bar. Any movement of the mouth or chin also moves the position of the eye, which means you will be chasing ocular structures with the microscope while trying to get a good look. Tell the patient to keep his or her teeth together and to breath through the nose.

What the Patient Needs to Know

- This instrument is a microscope used to magnify the structures of the eye.

- Please keep your chin in the cup with your teeth together and your forehead against the bar. Try not to lean back. The microscope comes close to your face but will not touch your eye.

- Sometimes the light is bright. Unless specifically told not to, you may blink at any time.

- Try to keep both eyes open.

- This is just a light, not a laser or a camera.

Adjust the height of the table and/or chair so the patient is not hunched over (table too low) or straining and stretching to reach the chin cup (table too high) (Figure 2-1A and 2-1B). If the table is too low, the patient will be uncomfortable. If the table is too high, the patient will be uncomfortable, plus he or she will tend to lean back out of the headrest. If the patient leans back, you will lose your focus. In addition, an uncomfortable patient tends to fidget. It is pretty tough to follow a tiny spot on the cornea at 40X if the patient is moving around! In most cases, the patient's back should be straight, the neck should be aligned with the back, and the patient may be leaning slightly forward over the hips. If the patient is leaning forward too much, ask him or her to slide forward a little, toward the edge of the chair seat.

Most slit lamp models have a mark or notch on the headrest bar. Adjust the height of the chin rest so that the patient's lateral canthus is aligned with the mark (Figure 2-2). When the patient is lined up properly, you will have the greatest latitude in moving the slit lamp.

Patients often do not know what to do with their hands when the table is placed over their lap. Show the patient how to grasp either side of the slit lamp table. This helps stabilize the patient (which is good for both the patient and the examiner) and the slit lamp. Sometimes the mechanisms to lock the table in place get stripped with use, and the table begins to drift even when locked. If the patient is holding the table on his or her side and you are leaning against the table on your side, such drifting can be kept to a minimum. In most cases, you should discourage the

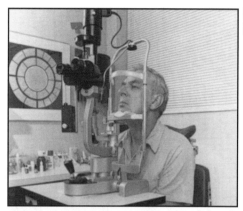

Figure 2-1A. The slit lamp is too high for the patient. (Photo by Mark Arrigoni.)

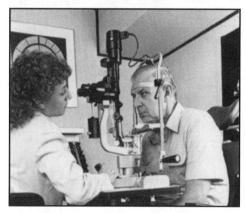

Figure 2-1B. The slit lamp is too low for the patient. (Photo by Mark Arrigoni.)

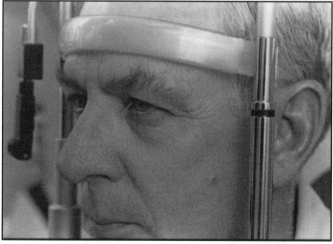

Figure 2-2. The instrument will have full range of movement if the eye is level with the marker. (Photo by Mark Arrigoni.)

patient from holding on to the sidebars of the headrest assembly. If the hands are placed too low, they might get pinched when you move the microscope forward. Some slit lamps have handles attached to the headrest unit for the patient to hold.

Patients come in different shapes and sizes, and positioning at the slit lamp may need to be modified a bit in certain cases. A large-busted woman may have difficulty leaning into the slit lamp. Once she is positioned, the slit lamp stage may not be able to move all the way forward, making

Figure 2-3. Attach a clip board to the bars as an adaptation for the large-breasted patient. (Photo by Val Sanders.)

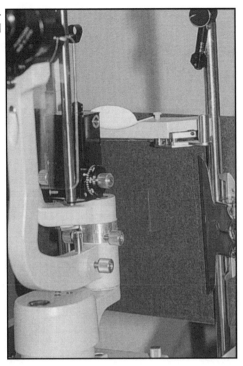

focusing impossible. In this situation, you may have to forfeit ideal patient alignment. Have the patient slide back into the exam chair as far as possible, then lean forward as far as possible into the slit lamp. By positioning her at such an angle, the bustline might be distanced far enough from the table. Another alternative is to attach a clipboard to the bars of the headrest assembly (Figure 2-3). (The patient may still need to be angled into the chin rest as described above.)

Children and other short persons may be better positioned by having the patient stand for the examination. The patient may be asked to stand on the floor just in front of the exam chair (Figure 2-4). A small child might be able to sit on a parent's lap for the slit lamp exam. This is convenient because it elevates the patient to a better height, plus the child feels safer. In addition, the parent can help stabilize the child.

In addition to positioning, a few other items will make examining children easier. This is one situation where you might tell the patient to hold on to the bars of the headrest assembly. Make sure that the child places his or her hands just under the chin rest so that the microscope will not pinch the hands when the stage is pushed forward.

Patient education before examining a child should be adapted as well. Pull the instrument forward. "See this? This is a fancy microscope for looking at your eye. This little cup is where your chin goes." Unless the child has been jumping all over the exam room and trying to play with all the equipment, invite him or her to touch the headrest part of the slit lamp. "This is sort of like a motorcycle, and this part [indicate chin rest, forehead strap] is the helmet. Can you put your chin right there? Good! Lean right up here like this. That's great! Now these are like the motorcycle's handles. [Put child's hands on bars under chin rest.] Hold on right there. Wonderful! Now here come the headlights...[start the exam]...Do you see a mouse in there? No? What about a rabbit? Here comes a turn! [Move the slit lamp to the other eye.] Do you see the mouse with this eye? Maybe a cat chased it away. Do you see a cat? Ride's over. Great job!"

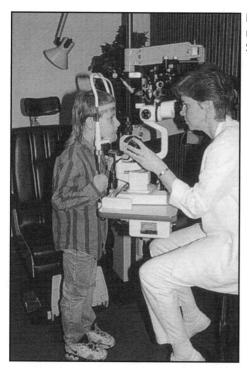

Figure 2-4. A short patient may be better able to reach the slit lamp when standing. (Photo by Val Sanders.)

An alternate child-patient education method is to demonstrate the use of the slit lamp on the parent before attempting to examine the child. You could allow the child to look at the parent's eye through the microscope, reinforcing the ideas: 1) this does not hurt, and 2) this is really neat. As with most testing on a child, decide before starting what information is the most important, and get that first. For example, if a child has a family history of congenital cataracts, examining the lens is the most important thing. So check the lens of each eye first. Then, if patient cooperation permits, check out the other structures. (This same strategy applies to a potentially uncooperative patient of any age.)

A wheelchair-bound patient presents another positioning difficulty. If your office does not have a wheelchair instrument stand, the best solution is to transfer the patient into the exam chair. This is not always possible. To examine a patient in a wheelchair, using a standard instrument stand, you may need to turn the exam chair so it is out of the way. If the armrests on the wheelchair come off, remove them, and the slit lamp should slide right over the patient's lap. In chairs where the armrests are not removable, the patient will have to lean forward a fair distance (Figure 2-5). See if the patient can slide forward a little in the chair. If the patient is weak, have an assistant help him or her lean forward into the chin rest. You might place pillows behind the patient to prop him or her. An extra assistant will probably be needed to hold the patient's head in position. This may be another situation where you should decide what is most important and examine that first, before the patient wears out.

Sometimes, getting the patient into position is not a problem, but other conditions may make modifications necessary. If the patient constantly chews or moves the mouth, you should drop the chin rest all the way down, out of the way. Have the patient lean into the forehead rest, without using the chin rest. You may need an assistant to help stabilize the patient's head, which may tend to drift down.

Examining a patient with head tremors can be challenging. Try having an assistant stabilize the patient's head from behind.

Figure 2-5. Positioning a patient in a wheelchair. (Photo by Val Sanders.)

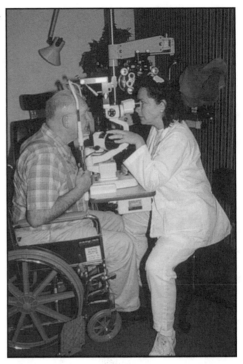

Patients with nystagmus have often learned that their vision is better if they hold their head in a certain position. This is because the jerking movements are quieter in a certain gaze. Before examining a patient with nystagmus, ask how he or she holds the head to see the best. Try to duplicate that position at the slit lamp. This may mean that the patient's head is turned instead of facing straight ahead or that you must drop the chin rest out of the way. In addition, encourage the patient to keep both eyes open at all times. Occluding one eye often makes the movements worse.

Occlusion may work in your favor, however, in the patient with strabismus. If the patient's eye turn is large enough to pull the eye out of alignment with the microscope, apply a patch to the other eye. Then ask the patient to look straight ahead.

A patient who is in pain can be very difficult to examine. Once it has been determined that the patient does not have a penetrating injury, a drop of anesthetic may be instilled, if the physician approves. Although the eye is then numb, the patient may still be photophobic. Stress the importance of the exam, assure the patient that you will use the dimmest light possible, and explain that you will do your best to be quick and thorough. Decide what information is most important, and examine that structure first. (In severe cases, a technician may want to defer the exam to the physician so that the patient will have to endure only one examination rather than two.)

Adjust Ocular Eyepieces

Like with many pieces of ophthalmic equipment, the first thing you should do before beginning the actual examination is adjust the eyepieces of the slit lamp oculars.

If you wear glasses, decide if you are going to wear them or remove them when you use the slit lamp. If you remove them, the oculars must be set to compensate for your refractive error. Whether you use the slit lamp with or without correction, you will be more comfortable if you

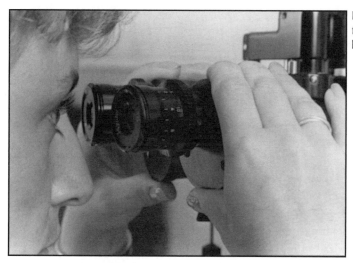

Figure 2-6. Setting the oculars for pupillary distance. (Photo by Mark Arrigoni.)

can eliminate your own accommodative response. This means using the most plus (or least minus) possible.

Tape a piece of white paper to the forehead bar. Set the oculars to the most plus position. Shine the wide open beam on the paper. Close the left eye, and slowly turn the right ocular toward minus. Stop as soon as the field is clear. Close the right eye and do the same with the left ocular. Do not keep turning once the field is clear. The focus may seem to get very slightly clearer, but you are now stimulating accommodation.

Some slit lamp manufacturers include a focusing test rod with the accessory kit. The rod is inserted into the hole used for the Hruby lens, with the black surface visible through the slit lamp. Then, the oculars are turned as described above. Each ocular should be set individually.

After you have done this a few times and found the ideal setting for your eyes, you can automatically set the oculars without sighting through them every time. Adjusting the eyepiece of the oculars before positioning the patient will reduce the amount of time that the patient must spend at the slit lamp, an important factor in some cases.

You will also need to set the pupillary distance (PD) of the oculars (Figure 2-6). This can be done quickly at the beginning of the exam. Firmly grasp the movable portion of the oculars and slide them in or out. If you see crescents on the outer edge, the PD is set too close. If crescents appear at the inner edge, the PD is too wide. There is nothing scientific about this; just slide the oculars until you have an unobstructed view with both eyes.

Power Up

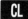

Before turning on the lamp, unlock the stage and move it to the forward left corner. Turn the illumination dial so that only a thin beam will appear when the instrument is turned on. (On some models, however, you cannot tell how wide the beam will be by just looking.) With the stage in this position and the beam turned down, the patient will not get a glaring light in the face when you switch the light on. Even if the beam is at full width, with the stage forward left, the light should fall to the side of the patient's face.

Figure 2-7. Set the transformer to the lowest or mid voltage setting. (Photo by Mark Arrigoni.)

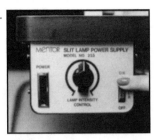

Turn the transformer on at the lowest or mid voltage setting (Figure 2-7). Using the lower settings extends the bulb's life. A sudden surge of higher-voltage power through a bulb can cause the bulb to blow. The lower setting is adequate for most examination purposes, anyway.

If nothing happens when you turn on the instrument you will need to play detective and figure out what is going on. Start with the most simple things and go from there:

- Is the slit beam misdirected (via scanning control ring or slit centering knob)?
- Is the slit beam closed?
- Is something obstructing the optical head?
- Is a filter halfway engaged?
- Is the main switch on? How about any secondary power switches?
- Is there a good connection between the transformer and lamp?
- Is there a good connection between the transformer and the power source?
- Is the instrument plugged in?
- Has the bulb blown?
- Has the fuse blown?
- Have you blown a circuit breaker?

If all of these items check out, refer to your instruction manual and call the manufacturer, if necessary.

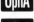

Fixation

Giving the patient something to look at while you examine him or her helps hold the eye steady. If your slit lamp has a fixation light, have the patient look at that (Figure 2-8). If you do not have a fixation device, you can ask the patient to look straight ahead at your ear or over your shoulder at a large letter or other target at the end of the room. (Remember that the target may be obscured at times as you swing the light source back and forth.) Encourage the patient to keep both eyes open and to blink now and then.

Magnification

It is a good idea to begin the examination at 6X or 10X magnification. You can move to 16X or more when you examine the cornea and internal structures and when you see some abnormality that warrants closer inspection. Remember that the higher the magnification setting, the more magnified the patient's movements become. A tiny flutter may be barely noticeable at 6X but take

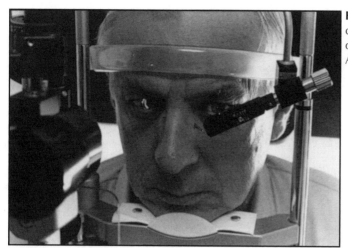

Figure 2-8. Using a fixation light can help reduce eye movement during the exam. (Photo by Mark Arrigoni.)

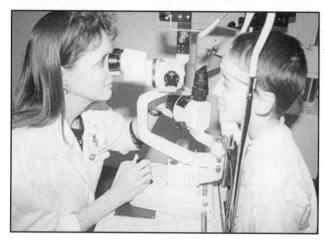

Figure 2-9. One hand manipulates the joystick, and the other hand operates the light source. (Photo by Val Sanders.)

your object of interest totally out of the field at 40X. Table 2-1 lists suggested magnifications for various parts of the slit lamp exam.

Manipulating the Light Source

The ideal examiner position is to have one hand on the light source and the other hand on the joystick (Figure 2-9). The hand on the light source can manipulate beam width, angle, and height usually at the same time.

Focusing

In a previous section, we instructed you to move the stage over to the forward left corner once the patient is positioned. If the beam is not narrow when the light is turned on, narrow it now. Angle the light at about 45 degrees. Move the stage to the right (keeping forward as much as possible without physically contacting the patient), allowing the beam to fall on the patient's face. If the beam is lower or higher than the eye, rotate the joystick (or the joystick ring) to make the beam level with the eye. Now, slide the stage right until the beam falls on the patient's temporal canthus of the right eye.

OptT
CL

Continued on page 28

TABLE 2-1

SLIT LAMP EXAMINATION

Suggested Power

6X or 10X	external (lids, conjunctiva), contact lenses
16X	angles, cornea, lens, foreign bodies, corneal abrasions
40X	corneal endothelium (described in text)

Beam Width

1 narrowest (Figure 2-10)	angles, cornea, anterior chamber
2 a bit wider (Figure 2-11)	cornea, lens, etc
3 a bit wider yet (Figure 2-12)	external, contact lenses
4 full width (Figure 2-13)	external, applanation tension (with blue filter)

Beam Height

full	most areas and structures
short (Figure 2-14)	checking anterior chamber for cells & flare

Color/Filter

white	most areas and structures
blue	(use fluorescein dye) applanation tensions, corneal staining, tear film, staining patterns of rigid contact lenses
green (red-free)	evaluating blood vessels, iron lines

Position (of light source)

R= right
L= left
C= center
degrees (given; indicated at base of illumination arm)

Stage (position)

R= right
L= left

Abbreviations

OD	right eye
OS	left eye
SCH	subconjunctival hemorrhage
AC	anterior chamber
SPK	superficial punctate keratopathy
PEE	punctate epithelial erosions
PSC	posterior subcapsular cataract
AT	applanation tension

Note: Unless contraindicated, fluorescein is instilled before slit lamp exam begins. Abnormalities are explained in Chapter 5.

Table 2-1 (continued)
SLIT LAMP EXAMINATION
Suggested Slit Lamp Exam Protocol

Settings	Area/Structure	Observe for

OD Lids (Figure 2-15)

Power: 10X		blepharospasm
Width: 2 to 4		collarettes
Height: full		coloboma
Color: white		crusting/matting
Position: R, sweep to L		discharge
Stage: L		edema (swelling)
		erythema
		growths
		lash loss
		lid closure
		lid lag
		lid position
		notching
		reflux
		trauma

OS Lids

Position: R, sweep to L		
Stage: R		

OD Conjunctiva, Episclera, Sclera (Figure 2-16)

Power: 10X to 16X		ciliary flush
Width: 2		color
Position: L, sweep to R		dryness
Stage: L		edema (chemosis)
		follicles
		foreign body
		growths
		injection
		leash vessels
		papillae
		pinguecula
		scleral show
		scleral thinning
		SCH
		trauma

OD Tear Film

Power: 10X to 16X		break up time
Width: 2		debris
Position: L, sweep to R		discharge
Stage: L		epiphora

OD Cornea (Figure 2-17)

Width: 2		abrasion
Position: L, sweep to R		arcus senilis
		dellen
		dystrophy

Table 2-1 (continued)
SLIT LAMP EXAMINATION
Suggested Slit Lamp Exam Protocol

Settings	Area/Structure	Observe for
	OD Cornea (Figure 2-17) (continued)	
		edema
		filaments
		foreign body
		ghost vessels
		guttata
		infiltrates
		iron lines
		keratitic precipitates
		keratitis
		keratopathy
		Krukenberg spindles
		opacities
		pannus
		phlyctenule
		pterygium
		rust ring
		scar
		stria/folds
		ulcer
		vascularization
	OD Corneal Staining	
Color: blue		abrasion
Position: L, sweep to R		bullae
		dendrites
		dry spots
		PEE/SPK
		stained areas
		tear film
		ulcer
	OD Temporal Angle (Figure 2-18)	
Power: 16X		AC depth
Width: 1		angle grade
Color: white		
Position: L, ~45°		
	OD Nasal Angle	
Position: R, ~45°		
	OD AC (Figure 2-19)	
Width: 1 to 2		hyphema
Position: L, sweep to R		hypopyon
		vitreous
Width: 1		cells
Height: small		flare
Position: L, sweep to R with		
vertical searching motions		

Table 2-1 (continued)
SLIT LAMP EXAMINATION
Suggested Slit Lamp Exam Protocol

Settings	Area/Structure	Observe for
	OD Iris/Pupil (Figure 2-20)	
Width: 2		atrophy
Height: full		coloboma
Position: L, sweep to R		iris detachment
		iris movement
		iris nevus
		iris strands
		laser iridotomy
		normal iris vessels
		peripheral iridectomy
		pigment dispersion
		pupil reaction
		pupil shape
		rubeosis
		sector iridectomy
		synechiae
	OD Lens (Figure 2-21)	
		cortical spoking
		nuclear sclerosis
		opacities
		PSC
		pseudoexfoliation
		subluxation
		vacuoles
	OD Intraocular Lens	
		capsule opacity
		capsulotomy
		location
		position
		precipitates
	OD Anterior Vitreous	
Position: L, sweep to R		clarity
		opacities
	OS Conjunctiva and Globe	
(repeat process using opposite directions)		
	AT, OD	
Power: 6 or 10X		
Height: full		
Width: full		
Color: blue		
Position: L, ~60°		
Stage: L		
	AT, OS	
Position: R		
Stage: R		

Figure 2-10. Thin vertical slit beam. (Reprinted with permission from *Ophthalmic Photography*, SLACK Incorporated. Photo by Steve Carlton.)

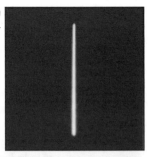

Figure 2-11. Slightly wider beam. (Photo by Val Sanders.)

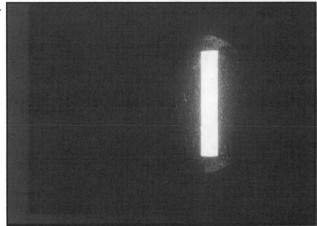

Figure 2-12. The beam is wider yet. (Photo by Val Sanders.)

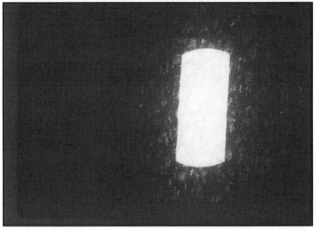

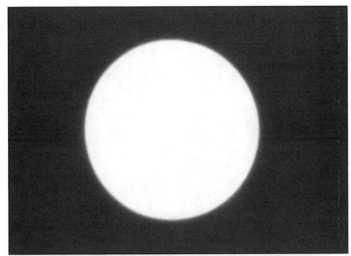

Figure 2-13. Wide open slit beam. (Reprinted with permission from *Ophthalmic Photography*, SLACK Incorporated. Photo by Steve Carlton.)

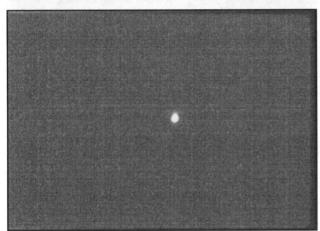

Figure 2-14. Pinpoint beam. (Photo by Val Sanders.)

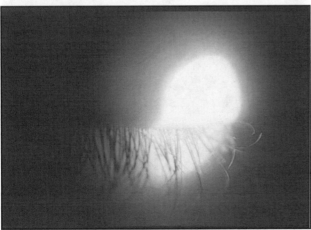

Figure 2-15. Lids, right eye. Moderately wide beam. (Photo by Val Sanders.)

Figure 2-16. Examining the temporal conjunctiva, episclera, and sclera. (Photo by Val Sanders.)

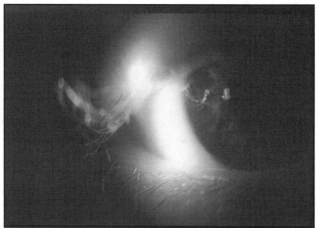

Figure 2-17. Cornea, right eye. (Photo by Val Sanders.)

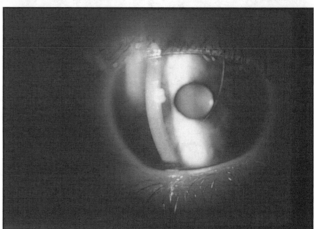

Figure 2-18. Evaluating the temporal angle, right eye. Notice the dark interval between the corneal section and the light reflection on the iris. Narrowest beam at full height. (Photo by Val Sanders.)

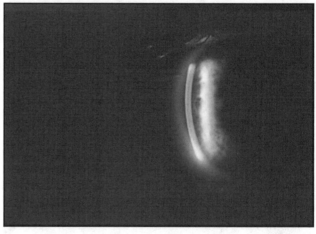

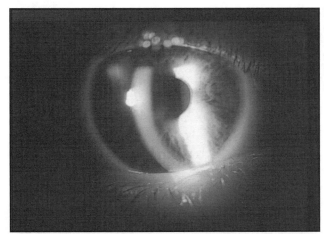

Figure 2-19. Examining the anterior chamber, right eye. Note that the beam is not sharply focused on either the cornea or the iris, indicating that it is focused on the anterior chamber. (Photo by Val Sanders.)

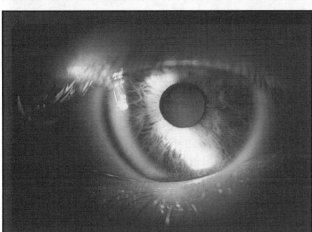

Figure 2-20. Iris and pupil, right eye. (Photo by Val Sanders.)

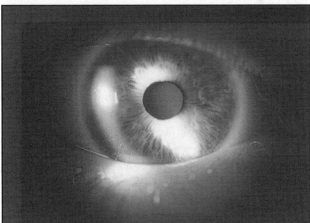

Figure 2-21. Right lens. (Photo by Val Sanders.)

Your initial act of focusing can be done one of two ways. First, you can look at the beam on the patient's eye from the side of the instrument. Slowly pull back on the joystick until you can see that the beam edges are sharp and crisp. Once the eye is grossly aligned, the examiner should look through the oculars and finetune the focus on whatever structure of the eye is being examined. If your initial line-up was good, only slight movements of the joystick will be necessary.

The second method of focusing is done while looking through the slit lamp the entire time. Since you have started with the stage all the way forward, you know that the only possible motion in order to focus is to pull back. Move the stage back slowly with the joystick until the eye is focused. This method is ideal for beginners because it avoids *searching* with the microscope (and the attending sensation of incompetence).

If the light is falling on the eye, yet you do not see anything when you look through the oculars, you will get to play detective again:

- Are the oculars set for your PD?
- Is the magnification dial clicked firmly into place?
- Is the slit image control/ring clicked into the straight-ahead position?

If you see an image through one ocular and not the other, check your PD and ocular focus. Also, recheck the ocular focus setting if the image from one eye seems fuzzy. If the slit beam does not coincide with the image centered in the microscope, check to see that the slit control/ring is in the straight-ahead position.

Staying focused is a matter of patient education and cooperation. Sometimes you will loose focus because the patient has leaned back. This may be a natural, protective gesture when something is coming right at the face. If this is the case, remind the patient to lean forward again, reassuring him or her that the instrument will not touch the face. Check the patient's position. If the patient is too low, it is difficult to stay against the forehead band. Raise the chair a little, and the head will tip back into the head rest.

Special Procedures

You can instill drops with the patient at the slit lamp. Just slide the stage all the way back, and have the patient look up. Pull the lower lid down and place the drop into the cul de sac.

If the patient has ptosis or an otherwise droopy upper lid, you may need to hold it up at the same time you are doing the examination. First, adjust the light angle and slit beam to the desired position. To hold up the patient's right upper lid, use your left thumb. Have the patient look down, place your thumb at the lid crease, then roll the thumb upward. This also rolls up the lid. Brace your thumb against the bone of the upper orbit, being careful not to place pressure on the globe. Brace the heel of your hand on the upright bar of the headrest assembly. Ask the patient to resume looking straight ahead. Keep your right hand on the joystick. Look through the instrument, and adjust your focus. Use the right hand to hold up the left lid.

If you must examine the underside of the upper lid, you will have to evert the lid (Figure 2-22). Pull the slit lamp stage all the way back, out of the way. (The patient remains positioned at the slit lamp.) Ask the patient to look down without closing the eyes. To evert the right upper lid, grasp the lashes with the left thumb and forefinger. Pull the lid gently outward. At the same time, place your right forefinger at the lid crease and push that part of the lid down. Then hold the everted lid in place with the left thumb, bracing the heel of your hand against the upright bar of the headrest assembly. The patient should continue looking down. Move your right hand to the joystick, and slide the stage forward so the beam falls on

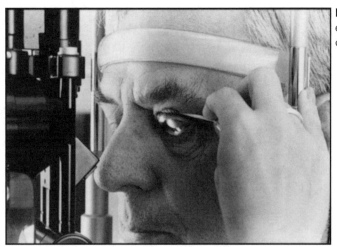

Figure 2-22. The upper lid can be everted using a cotton-tipped applicator. (Photo by Mark Arrigoni.)

the lid. Look through the instrument, adjusting your focus. To un-evert the lid, just let go and tell the patient to look up.

The upper lid can also be everted over the stick of a cotton swab. Pull the slit lamp stage all the way back, out of the way. (The patient remains positioned at the slit lamp.) Ask the patient to look down without closing the eyes. Gently place the stick across the lid crease using the left hand. With the right thumb and forefinger, grasp the lashes, pulling out and up while pressing down with the stick. The lid should flip. Continue to hold the stick with the left hand while you focus with the right. Brace the hand against the upright of the headrest assembly, and examine as outlined above. The lid will unevert when the patient looks up.

Getting Your Bearings

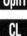

Knowing anatomical planes and directions will help you in orienting yourself as well as in describing things during the documentation phase of the exam (Figure 2-23). Divisions of the globe itself are described in Chapter 3. Ocular landmarks and dimensions are shown in Figure 2-24.

Protocol and Documentation

It is important to develop your own slit lamp examination protocol. Performing the exam the same way, in the same order, on every patient, will increase the quality of your examination by ensuring that nothing is missed. Table 2-1 is a typical protocol. This protocol might be modified depending on the patient and the situation. For example, if the patient is uncooperative, select the structures that are most vital and examine them first. In addition, each examiner may modify this plan to suit him- or herself. For example, some might prefer to completely examine the right eye before moving to the left rather than the method suggested here.

It is customary to position the light housing on the left when examining structures to the (examiner's) left of the midline. When you reach the midline, move the light to the right side. Examine the midline area again; then continue by checking the structures to the right.

Figure 2-23. Anatomical directions. (Reprinted with permission from *Medical Sciences for the Ophthalmic Assistant*, SLACK Incorporated.)

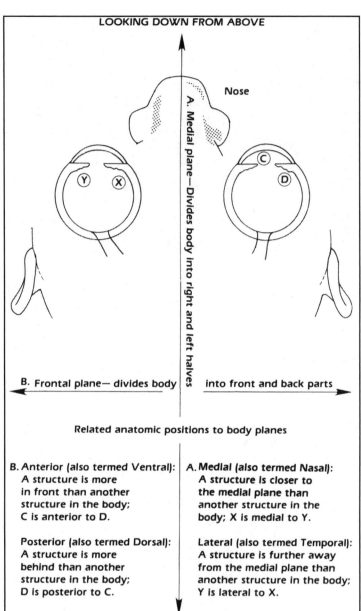

LOOKING DOWN FROM ABOVE

Nose

A. Medial plane—Divides body into right and left halves

B. Frontal plane— divides body | into front and back parts

Related anatomic positions to body planes

B. Anterior (also termed Ventral):
A structure is more
in front than another
structure in the body;
C is anterior to D.

Posterior (also termed Dorsal):
A structure is more
behind than another
structure in the body;
D is posterior to C.

A. Medial (also termed Nasal):
A structure is closer to
the medial plane than
another structure in the
body; X is medial to Y.

Lateral (also termed Temporal):
A structure is further away
from the medial plane than
another structure in the body;
Y is lateral to X.

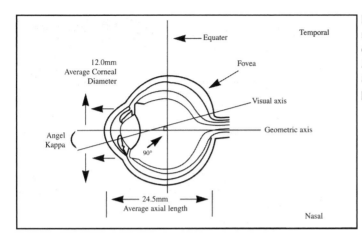

Figure 2-24. Schematic of common ocular landmarks and dimensions. (Modified from *Medical Sciences for the Ophthalmic Assistant*, SLACK Incorporated.)

Documentation is the last step of the slit lamp exam. It is not enough to look at the eye; you must write down what you see, even if it is normal. Never underestimate the importance of accurate, legible notations in the patient's chart. (Remember these axioms: "If it's not in the chart, it wasn't done. If it's not readable, it's not in the chart.") Such notes may be the only thing that keeps you and/or your employer from being sued.

It is important to note findings, not diagnoses. For example, write, "3+ lash crusting, 2+ lid edema, 2+ lash loss" instead of "blepharitis." Blepharitis is a diagnosis and belongs in the physician's assessment. For more on this topic, see Chapter 5. The subjective grading system is discussed in that chapter, as well.

In cases where abnormalities are expected yet not found, you may record negative information. For example, the patient has diabetes, so you carefully examine the iris for abnormal blood vessels (rubeosis). Finding none, record, "No iris rubeosis."

If abbreviations are used, they should be standardized and written down for the office. This small bit of effort might also save you in court. Documentation advocates are fond of saying that the abbreviation WNL (which is supposed to mean "within normal limits") means "we never looked." Do not fall into sloppy documentation habits. It is better to write out the words "clear" or "normal." Do not neglect to note a normal finding just because it is normal.

Documentation of specific structures and findings is discussed in Chapters 3 and 5.

Chapter 3

A Magnified Tour of the Normal Eye

KEY POINTS

- An appreciation of what is normal is necessary before one can identify that which is abnormal.

- Documenting that a structure is normal is just as important as notating irregularities.

- There are variations of normal that you will learn as you continue to examine eyes with the slit lamp.

Before one can appreciate something that is abnormal, one must be thoroughly acquainted with "normal." By studying normal eyes, you will soon learn to spot anything unusual. This chapter gives a slit lamp view of the normal eye. Granted, there are variations of normal. Abnormalities that are mentioned in this chapter will be explained more fully in Chapter 5.

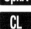

External Ocular Adnexa

By definition, the ocular adnexa includes the lids, lacrimal system, orbit, and surrounding tissue (Figure 3-1). We will explore only those structures visible with the slit lamp. These external structures are screened with a moderately wide or full beam and 6X or 10X magnification. A beam angle of about 45 degrees is good, with the light directed from the left to examine the patient's lateral right eye and medial left eye, and directed from the right to examine the patient's lateral left eye and medial right eye. The power can be increased to study any abnormalities (see Chapter 5). While we have listed documentation for each eyelid structure, the single notation *lids clear* is often used to refer to the lids as a whole.

Eyebrows

The eyebrow separates the upper lid from the forehead by several rows of short hairs. Brow color is generally the same as hair color. The brows may become gray or white with age.
Documentation: brows clear

Dermis (Skin)

The skin covering the lids is thin, elastic, loose, and nearly hairless. Except for wrinkles, the skin should be smooth and its color should match the individual's overall skin tone. The crease in the upper lid represents the insertion point of the levator muscle. The upper lid ends at the eyebrow, while the lower lid blends into the cheek.
Documentation: lids clear; color normal

Medial and Lateral Canthi

The canthi are the corners of the eye where the upper and lower lids meet. The lateral canthus (toward the ear) forms a 30 to 40 degree angle and should hug tightly against the globe. The medial canthus (next to the nose) is more open and rounded and may be covered by a fold of skin in some individuals. This fold is called the epicanthus and is normal in individuals of Asian descent. Infants of any race may exhibit an epicanthus, but in this case, the fold usually disappears as the child grows. It is also seen in individuals with Down Syndrome.
Documentation: canthi normal; epicanthus present/absent

Lid Margin

The lid margin forms a small 2.00 mm "shelf" between the rows of lashes and where the lid touches the globe. The length of the lid margin from canthus to canthus is 25.00 to 30.00 mm. There should not be any lashes growing from the lid margin itself. The lid margin should be clean, smooth, and flesh-toned or slightly paler. The gray line, which is a faint line that runs down the center of the lid margin, may be visible. Tiny oil glands in the lids open onto the lid margin. These

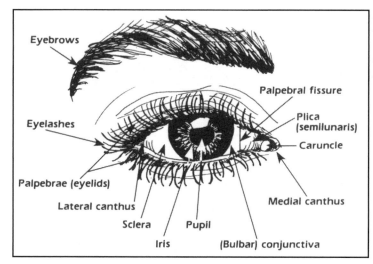

Figure 3-1. The external eye. (Reprinted with permission from *Medical Sciences for the Ophthalmic Assistant*, SLACK Incorporated.)

openings are visible under higher magnifications. If the glands are full of oil, tiny droplets (meibomian plugs) may appear on the lid margin. The lid margin might be slightly moist, but any moisture should be clear (ie, tears). The inner edge should "hug" (approximate) the eyeball.
Documentation: margins smooth; approximate globe

Eyelashes

The eyelashes are cilia (fine hairs) that grow from follicles at the lid margins. Five to 6 irregular rows are found on the upper lid and 3 to 4 rows on the lower. There are about 100 to 150 lashes on the upper lid, and the lower lid has 50 to 75. Lashes are thicker, more numerous, and more curled in childhood. Each cilia should curve outward, away from the globe. There should be no obvious gaps where cilia are missing. The base of each lash should cleanly enter the skin. There may be some shorter young lashes, but each lash should be tapered at the end (ie, not broken off). The lashes of the upper lid are generally longer than those of the lower lid. Lashes are often darker than the hair color and do not whiten with age. The lashes are very sensitive, and touching them will cause the patient to blink.
Documentation: lashes normal

Puncta

The puncta are tiny openings (averaging 0.30 mm), one in the upper lid and one in the lower, found about 2.00 to 4.00 mm temporal to the medial canthus. In the normal eye, the lids roll in onto the globe so that the puncta are in contact with the eye. To view the punctum with the microscope, you will have to roll the lid out.
Documentation: puncta open; approximate globe

Caruncle

The caruncle is a yellowish, pink, or flesh-toned mound of tissue that lies against the globe at the medial canthus. It contains sweat and oil glands (not visible) and fine, colorless hairs that grow outward toward the nose.
Documentation: caruncle normal

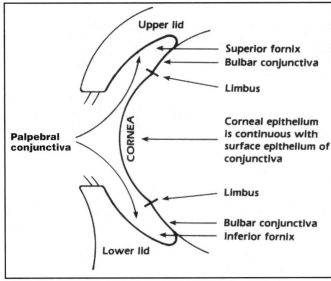

Figure 3-2. Schematic cross-section of conjunctival topography. (Reprinted with permission from *Medical Sciences for the Ophthalmic Assistant,* SLACK Incorporated.)

Plica Semilunaris

The plica is a pale half-moon shaped fold of tissue just lateral to the caruncle. It represents the junction of the bulbar conjunctiva (described below) and muscle tissue. It is loosely attached, and when the patient abducts the eye, you can see the plica stretch and unfold.
Documentation: plica normal

Palpebral Conjunctiva

The inside of the lids is lined with a mucous membrane called the palpebral conjunctiva (Figure 3-2). This membrane is tightly adherent to the underlying tissue. The palpebral conjunctiva of the lower lid may be easily examined by pulling the lid down. To see under the upper lid, you will have to evert the lid (see Chapter 2). The palpebral conjunctiva is normally pale pink and may be slightly bumpy. (See Chapter 5 regarding follicles and papillae, which are abnormalities.) You might see a few fine yellow lines running just underneath the surface. These are meibomian glands.
Documentation: palpebral conjunctiva clear

Bulbar Conjunctiva

The bulbar conjunctiva is a thin mucous membrane that lies over the globe up to the point of the limbus. After the limbus, only the very surface cells (epithelium) of the conjunctiva blend into the corneal epithelium. It is normally clear in caucasians. The conjunctiva of dark-skinned individuals may be totally or partially pigmented. While the palpebral conjunctiva that lines the lids is tightly anchored to the tissue beneath, the bulbar conjunctiva is loose and moveable. The bulbar conjunctiva contains blood vessels, which normally are so tiny that they are nearly transparent. The bulbar conjunctiva also contains accessory glands that are not visible. The bulbar conjunctiva joins with the palpebral conjunctiva in the fornix. (When the word *conjunctiva* is used without designating bulbar or palpebral, the bulbar conjunctiva is usually what is being referred to.)

Rose bengal dye is used to detect dead (devitalized) or degenerated conjunctival and/or corneal epithelial cells. Thirty seconds after the dye is instilled, the cul de sac (inferior fornix) is gently irrigated. The eye is then viewed at the slit lamp under white light. In the normal, healthy eye, there will be no stained areas.

Documentation: conjunctiva clear without injection; no stain

Fornix

The pocket under the lids where the palpebral and bulbar conjunctiva join is called the fornix. The inferior fornix is examined by simply pulling down the lower lid while the patient looks up. The superior fornix is difficult to examine thoroughly because it is so deep. Pull the patient's upper lid up as far as possible while the patient looks down. If you can elevate the upper lid far enough to leave a gap between the lid margin and the globe, you may be able to see into the pocket a little farther. (If this is not adequate, you may have to abandon the slit lamp, double evert the lid, and use a pen light and loupes.)

Documentation: fornices clear

Lid Position

The normal lid margin will contact the globe without any gaps (except at the medial canthus). The lids should also be positioned so that the cilia are directed outward, away from the eyeball. When the patient closes his or her eye, the lids should contact each other completely without any gaps. When open, the lid should completely uncover the pupil. When the eye is fully opened, a small portion of the superior and inferior cornea (1.00 to 2.00 mm) should still be covered. When the patient looks up or down, the upper lid should follow the globe without hesitation.

Documentation: lid position normal

The Blink

Blinking serves to swab tears over the eye to keep the external globe moist and free of foreign material. The upper and lower lids should glide freely over the globe and meet without any gaps during each blink. The average blink rate is every 3 to 6 seconds.

Documentation: complete blink; blink rate ___

External Eye

Tear Film

The tear film serves to keep the external globe moist as well as to wash debris and foreign matter away. The tear film is composed of three layers: mucin, water, and oil. Each component is made by various glands that are not visible with the slit lamp. The three layers are not individually identifiable if present in proper proportions.

Each blink acts to spread the tears over the eye, a phenomenon that can be seen with the slit lamp. The pumping action of the blink moves the tears toward the medial canthus, where they gather into the lacrimal lake. Here the tears pool slightly before draining through the puncta. If the tear film is adequate, the entire visible external eye should be evenly coated with each blink.

The tears also lubricate each blink, enabling the lids to move smoothly over the eye without pulling on the conjunctiva.

The use of rose bengal dye (described above) is actually an evaluation of the cells that create the tear film's mucin layer. If no staining is present, the tear film is considered adequate.

Fluorescein dye is also used to evaluate tear film stability. After the dye is instilled, the eye is examined with the slit lamp using the cobalt blue filter. A thin beam is used to prevent evaporation of the tears due to heat from the light. The patient is asked first to blink, then to open the lids wide while looking straight ahead. (The lids are not physically held apart.) The examiner counts the number of seconds from the blink until the tear film begins to break up, revealing black spots where the film is drying. This is known as the tear break up time (BUT). If normal, the dyed tear film should remain cohesive for at least 15 seconds.

Documentation: tear film clear and adequate; BUT = ___ seconds

Episclera and Sclera

The episclera lies between the bulbar conjunctiva and the sclera. It is a layer of thin, fine connective tissue that contains blood vessels which nourish the sclera. Like the conjunctiva, the episclera is loose and elastic. Its larger blood vessels differ from those of the conjunctiva in that they lie deeper and are not mobile.

The sclera is the "white" of the eye. It is composed of tough elastic tissue similar to cartilage. Surprisingly, the tissue of the sclera is the same type of tissue that makes up the cornea. Like the cornea, the sclera is avascular. The fibers of the sclera, however, are arranged in an irregular pattern. In addition, the sclera is a hydrated tissue. These two factors are why the sclera is opaque and the cornea is clear. When the sclera becomes dehydrated, it turns clear. It is normal for the sclera of children to have a bluish tint, but this would be abnormal in an adult. Persons of any race (but especially those with darker skin) may have pigmented spots on the sclera that are normal for that individual. Such lesions should be noted, however, as they may indicate abnormal findings. Sometimes, a nerve loop might be visible on the sclera. This looks like a fine, blackish-silver filament. They are more common nasally and are actually loops of the long ciliary nerve.

Documentation: the eye is white

Limbus

The limbus is a 1.00 mm wide gray, semitransparent zone that represents the junction between the sclera and the cornea. With the slit lamp, you may be able to see tiny blood vessels (capillaries) that run from the limbus just into the cornea. A key characteristic of these normal vessels is that they loop back into the limbus.

Documentation: limbus normal

Cornea

The slit lamp was developed with the cornea in mind. The cornea is a curved transparent structure, much like the crystal on a watch. If you look at a watch glass while light is hitting its face straight on, the glass appears shiny and smooth. However if you view the glass with the light source coming from the side, at an angle, you can see scratches and pits. The slit lamp allows us to direct light onto the cornea from an angle. Use a full height, narrow beam at about 45 degrees, switching sides when you cross the midline. Before finishing the exam, align the lamp with the

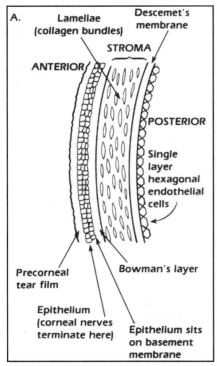

Figure 3-3A. Histologic cross-section of cornea.

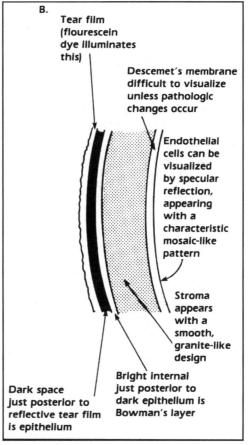

Figure 3-3B. Optic section of cornea as it appears under the slit lamp. (Reprinted with permission from *Medical Sciences for the Ophthalmic Assistant*, SLACK Incorporated.)

microscope so it is shining straight into the eye. The light will be reflected off of the lens and shine into the cornea from behind. This will cause the cornea to light up. Regardless of the light direction, etc, the cornea should be smooth and clear. While 6X or 10X magnification may be adequate to quickly screen the cornea, it is best observed with 16X.

The average adult cornea is about 11.50 mm across. It is thicker at the limbus (0.65 mm) and thinner in the center (0.54 mm). (Use a very thin slit to compare the thickness of the center to that of the edge.) Because the cornea is curved more steeply than the eyeball, it protrudes somewhat like a dome. When the patient looks down, the contour of the lower lid should indicate that the corneal curvature is smooth (ie, not pointed or conelike).

We mentioned above that the cornea and sclera are composed of the same type of fibers. However, while the fibers in the sclera run haphazardly, the corneal fibers are arranged in organized layers (lamellar bundles) like a lattice. Also, the cornea is dehydrated and avascular. These three factors contribute to the cornea's clarity.

The cornea is made up of five layers: epithelium, Bowman's membrane, stroma, Descemet's membrane, and endothelium (Figure 3-3A and 3-3B). The two membranes are slightly more reflective (and thus appear brighter) than the stroma. The epithelium and endothelium appear slightly darker than the stroma.

The cornea as a whole should be clear. The surface should be smooth, shiny, and tear-covered. The epithelium is about five cell-layers thick. Individual cells are not visible with the slit lamp. Fluorescein dye and the cobalt blue filter of the slit lamp are often used to evaluate the epithelium. In the normal epithelium, where there are no breaks, the fluorescein will wash over the surface uniformly. Rose bengal, described above, can also be used to detect dead or devitalized cells in the corneal epithelium. The normal, healthy cornea will not show any staining. The epithelium can regenerate itself and, thus, does not scar.

The basement (anchoring) membrane of the epithelium and Bowman's membrane are so thin that they are seen as one. Using a thin beam directed at about a 45-degree angle, these membranes appear as a thin bright line just beneath the darker epithelium.

The stromal layer comprises about 90% of the corneal structure. Sometimes you can see a few fine white threadlike filaments in the stroma, extending radially from the limbus but stopping before they reach the cornea's center. These are nerve fibers.

Descemet's membrane is a thin elastic layer that is stretched, kept taut by the force of the eye's internal pressure. It is not really visible unless something goes wrong. Then the membrane looses its tautness and wrinkles up (more on this in Chapter 4). In the normal cornea, it should not be distinct.

The corneal endothelium is a single cell layer thick. It should be smooth and clear. Direct a moderate width beam onto the cornea (at about 55 degrees) so that the reflection of light off of the epithelium dazzles you. Then move the light a little to the side and look next to it, at the reflection from the endothelial surface, and you can see the image of the cells. Use the highest magnification available.

Documentation: cornea clear, no stain

Anterior Segment

By convention, anterior segment refers to the eye's interior from the lens forward (Figure 3-4). Posterior segment indicates structures behind the lens. This is somewhat different from the terms anterior and posterior *chambers*, where the anterior chamber is between the iris and the cornea, and the posterior chamber is between the iris and the lens. (The anterior and posterior chambers are both part of the anterior segment.)

Anterior Chamber, Aqueous, and Angle

The anterior chamber of the eye is filled with a clear fluid called aqueous. The normal anterior chamber is optically empty.

The aqueous that fills the anterior chamber is constantly being formed and drained out. The aqueous drainage area is found in the angle, the area formed where the posterior corneal surface

meets the anterior iris root. (The angle itself cannot be viewed directly unless a gonio lens is used.) This dynamic creates a pressure within the eye, the IOP. Average IOP is around 15, ranging from 8 to 21. (Opinions vary as to what is *normal*.) IOP is measured using a tonometer, which may be attached to the slit lamp. If the IOP is abnormally high and continues to be high, the optic nerve may be damaged, which, in turn, can reduce the visual field. This condition is called glaucoma.

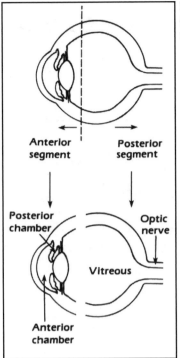

Figure 3-4. The anterior and posterior segments of the globe. (Reprinted with permission from *Medical Sciences for the Ophthalmic Assistant,* SLACK Incorporated.)

The depth of the anterior chamber is clinically significant. In a shallow chamber, the dilated iris may bunch up and block off the angle. This covers the aqueous drainage system, and the pressure of the stagnant (and continually forming) aqueous begins to build up. The pressure causes corneal edema (swelling that clouds the cornea), blurred vision (secondary to the edema), redness, pain, and optic nerve damage. This entire scenario is called angle closure glaucoma or a glaucoma attack. The likelihood of angle closure is related to the depth of the anterior chamber. If the chamber is deep, angle closure is unlikely to occur. Myopes, with their longer eyeballs, generally have a deep anterior chamber. The shorter eye of a hyperope is more likely to be shallow.

Estimating the depth of the anterior chamber is an important aspect of the slit lamp exam. To evaluate the chamber depth of the right eye, turn the lamp so that the light is coming at the temporal limbus at an angle of 60 degrees (Figure 3-5A). Change the slit to its most narrow setting, and direct the beam onto the cornea, just barely to the right of the limbus. You should see three things: the beam of light sharply focused on the cornea in a thin slit, the light falling on the iris (unfocused), and a dark interval in between (Figure 3-5B). The dark interval is the area of interest, as it represents the chamber's depth. If this shadow is one-quarter to one-half the width of the illuminated corneal section, the angle is open. If the dark section is less than one-quarter the width of the corneal beam, the chamber is narrow. If there is no dark interval (ie, the corneal and iris beams meet), the angle is extremely narrow or closed. The chamber is graded from 1 to 4 or labeled as closed, open, shallow, or moderate. (See Chapter 5 regarding subjective grading.) The nasal angle should be checked as well by swinging the beam to the right. The left eye is examined in the same way.

Documentation: anterior chamber deep and clear, angles open, grade 4

Figure 3-5A. Overhead schematic of angle estimation. (Drawing by Edmund Pett.)

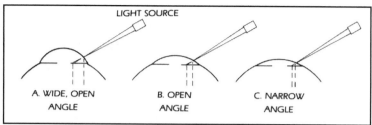

Figure 3-5B. Straight-on view of estimating chamber depth with the slit lamp. (Reprinted with permission from *Medical Sciences for the Ophthalmic Assistant*, SLACK Incorporated.)

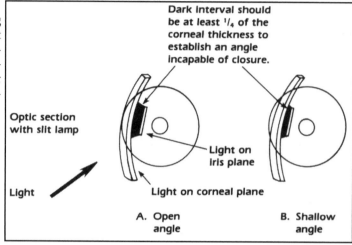

Anterior Chamber Intraocular Lens

When a cataract (cloudy lens) is removed, an intraocular lens (IOL) implant is usually placed inside the eye to focus incoming light. In current cataract surgical technique, the IOL generally is inserted behind the iris. Occasionally, certain cases necessitate IOL placement in front of the iris or in the anterior chamber. Anterior chamber IOLs were used more in the earlier years of implants but are still seen.

One of the most important concerns with an anterior chamber IOL is how it is held in place. You will be able to see posts, clips, or haptics (legs). Posts or clips should firmly anchor the IOL into the pupil. (An iris-fixed IOL that has posts or clips should *not* be dilated. The implant is held in place by the pupil; dilation of the eye may cause dislocation of the IOL.) Haptics should not dig into the cornea or angle. The optic might be round or rectangular. Regardless of shape, it should be even with the iris plane. The lens should also be centered over the pupil opening. *Documentation (if AC IOL is present): AC IOL clear and in place*

Iris

The iris is actually two muscles (Figure 3-6) whose fibers are easily visible with the slit lamp. The outer dilator muscle acts to open the pupil, and the inner sphincter muscle acts to constrict it. The colarette is a jagged area that represents the junction of these two muscles. The iris folds up and expands like an accordion, so it is normal to see ridges and crypts in it. The iris is a highly vascular tissue, but usually blood vessels are not visible unless the patient has very light colored irides. The important features of these vessels are that they follow the muscle fibers and do not branch out of this plane and that they are found within the fiber layer, rather than overlying

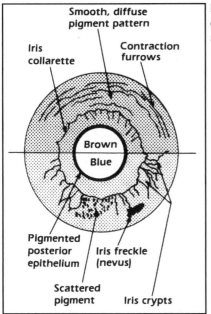

Figure 3-6. External view of a brown or blue iris. (Reprinted with permission from *Medical Sciences for the Ophthalmic Assistant,* SLACK Incorporated.)

the surface of the iris. (We will discuss the appearance of abnormal vessels in Chapter 5.) When you direct the beam straight-on and directly through the pupil, the pupil should light up, but light should not shine back through any part of the normal iris. There should be no movement of the iris except for changes in pupil size. The periphery of the iris should be attached at the angle.

There are many variations of normal regarding iris color, which may range from brown to green to blue to gray. Flecks of pigment may be scattered over the iris surface. The back of the iris is highly pigmented, which helps keep peripheral light from entering the eye. This layer sometimes wraps around the pupillary margin slightly and may appear as a dark frill. The irides should both be approximately the same color, pattern, and texture. The color should remain fairly constant throughout life.

Irides: blue (or whatever color) OU; clear

Pupil

The pupil is a round opening in the iris. While pupillary function is not evaluated with the slit lamp alone as a general rule, the undilated pupil should react by immediately getting smaller when the light of the slit lamp hits it. You may see pulsing movements of the pupil (hippus). If there was no pupillary reaction when the eyes were tested with a penlight, it is important to note whether or not they react to the brighter slit lamp light. The pupils are usually larger in young children and smaller in older adults. The size and reaction of the two pupils should be about equal.

Documentation: pupils round, reactive

Lens

The lens of the eye lies behind the pupil and acts to focus incoming light. It is a biconvex structure supported by tiny ligaments called zonules. The zonules are anchored in the ciliary muscle at the posterior base of the iris. The lens is about 9.00 to 10.00 mm in diameter and 4.00 mm thick.

The lens is best seen when the eye is dilated. However, even in dilation, the edges of the lens and the zonules will not be visible. The lens should be centrally located, and no movement should be detected. When you direct the beam straight-on and directly through the pupil, the lens should light up evenly without any opacities.

The lens is encased in an elastic envelope or capsule. The innermost heart of the lens is the nucleus. The outer material is the cortex. The normal lens is clear (a silvery-gray color) and avascular. During life, the lens lays down more layers of fibers with only a slight increase in size. As this happens, the material in the nucleus becomes compacted. Because the different layers have different indices of refraction, there is a subtle visual difference between them. These differences become more noticeable with age. There are two Y-shaped fissures (also called Y-sutures) in the nucleus of the lens, representing places where fibers meet. The first Y is upright, and the second Y is inverted. In an adult, the fissures may look like a star.

Documentation: lens clear

Posterior Chamber Intraocular Lens Implant

As mentioned above, most IOLs are placed into the posterior chamber, behind the pupil. Unless the pupil is dilated, you probably will not be able to see the haptics. (The haptics look like blue nylon fish line.) Only the center of the IOL's optic should be visible through the normal (undilated) pupil. The entire lens assembly should be in the posterior chamber, and the optic should be on a level plane with the iris.

Documentation (if PC IOL is present): PC IOL clear and in place

Posterior Lens Capsule

When a cataract is removed, the posterior lens capsule is often left in place to support a posterior IOL. If it is clear, as it should be, you may barely be able to see it. When you direct the beam straight-on and directly through the pupil, the capsule should light up evenly without any opacities or irregularities.

Documentation: capsule clear

Posterior Segment

Anterior Vitreous Face

The vitreous is a jellylike substance that fills the posterior segment of the eye. It is normally clear and avascular. There is a slight depression in the anterior vitreous face, creating a small space between it and the posterior lens capsule. Without using special lenses or attachments, the central portion of the anterior vitreous is the only posterior segment structure that can be seen with the slit lamp. This is easier, and the size of the visible area is increased, if the pupil is dilated.

Documentation: anterior vitreous clear

Chapter 4

Illumination Techniques

- The slit lamp exam is dynamic; the observer uses multiple types of illumination simultaneously.

- The three main categories of illumination are diffuse, direct, and indirect.

- Diffuse illumination provides an even light over the entire ocular surface.

- With direct illumination techniques, the light is shone directly onto the area or structure of interest.

- With indirect illumination methods, the object of interest is illuminated by light that is reflected off of another structure.

The usefulness of the slit lamp is a product of the illumination source (and its capabilities) and the microscope. The instrument is designed so that the beam is maximally focused at the same point where the microscope is focused. Various methods of illumination provide different ways of looking at tissues and abnormalities (Figures 4-1A and 4-1B). In previous chapters, we have merely told you what angle and slit characteristics to use when examining the eye. It is entirely possible to learn how best to view the structures without knowing the name of the type of illumination you are using. In this chapter, however, we will explore the various types of illumination and their uses for those who wish to delve further into the potential of the slit lamp.

Diffuse Illumination

In diffuse illumination, light is spread evenly over the entire observed surface (Figure 4-2). Diffuse illumination is most often used in slit lamp photography. However, it is still a good starting point for an examination, permitting a gross survey of the eye (especially the skin).

For an overall view, the beam is opened all the way. Direct the light onto the eye at a 45 degree angle. The microscope is directed straight ahead. If you do not have a neutral density filter (a frosted piece of plastic or ground glass that fits over or in front of the illuminator, also called a diffuser) on your instrument, decrease the illumination intensity. Use the least amount of magnification available (6X or 10X). The cobalt blue and red-free filters also act as diffusers, but white light is generally used for this technique.

Observe: eyelids, lashes, conjunctiva, sclera, pattern of redness, iris, pupil, gross pathology, and media opacities

Direct Illumination Techniques

Direct illumination is used for direct inspection of specific structures. It is especially useful in determining the depth of abnormalities. In these techniques, the light is directed at a specific object.

Beam

This illumination method is perhaps the best known and most used for observing the configuration and densities of opacities, lesions, and other abnormalities. It is important to note, however, that this illumination method may actually obscure certain details. Therefore, it must be used in conjunction with indirect techniques (especially for subtle corneal detail). Sweep the cornea or other structures with a narrow full-length beam (Figures 4-3A and 4-3B). The microscope is usually directed straight ahead but may also be moved to an angle opposite the illuminator. The greater the angle between the illuminator and the microscope, the greater the width of the illuminated section. A very narrow beam (optical section) directed onto the cornea can be used to evaluate corneal shape, elevation, and thickness. Such details are important when evaluating dellen or bullae.

Observe: cornea, iris, lens, vitreous

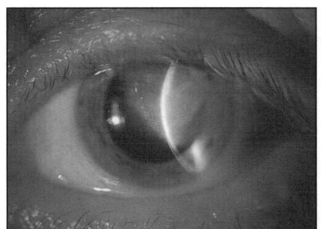

Figure 4-1A. A corneal opacity viewed under proximal illumination... (Photo by Val Sanders.)

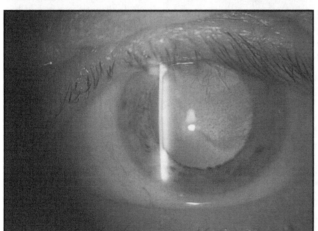

Figure 4-1B. ...and under direct iris retroillumination. Note that blood vessels are now visible. (Photo by Val Sanders.)

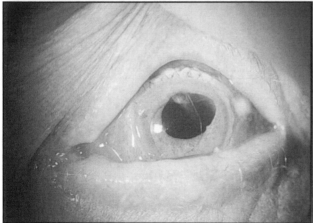

Figure 4-2. Diffuse illumination. (Photo by Val Sanders.)

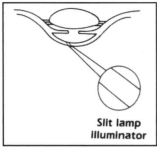

Figure 4-3A. Schematic of beam illumination. (Reprinted with permission from *Ophthalmic Photography*, SLACK Incorporated.)

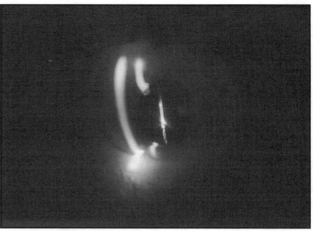

Figure 4-3B. Example of beam illumination (lens capsule). (Photo by Val Sanders.)

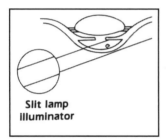

Figure 4-4A. Schematic of tangential illumination. (Reprinted with permission from *Ophthalmic Photography*, SLACK Incorporated.)

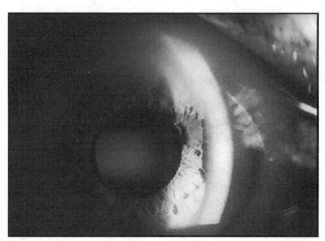

Figure 4-4B. Example of tangential illumination (iris). (Photo by Val Sanders.)

Tangential Illumination

This technique is used to observe surface texture. When a light is directed straight at an object, the view is rather flat. Tangential light (projected from an oblique angle) creates shadows, which highlight surface irregularities much the way that shading gives depth to drawings. Use a medium-wide beam of moderate height, and swing the slit lamp arm to the side at an oblique angle (almost parallel to the structure being viewed). The microscope is pointing straight ahead. The beam will sweep tangentially across the cornea, iris, or lens surface (Figures 4-4A and 4-4B). Magnifications of 10X, 16X, or 25X are used. If the iris is the structure of interest, it is best viewed without dilation. If you are looking for details on the cornea or lens, dilation is preferred because this creates a dark background against which to view those structures.

Observe: anterior and posterior cornea, iris, anterior lens (especially useful for viewing pseudoexfoliation)

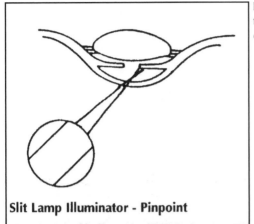

Slit Lamp Illuminator - Pinpoint

Figure 4-5A. Schematic of pinpoint (conical section) illumination. (Adapted with permission from *Ophthalmic Photography*, SLACK Incorporated.)

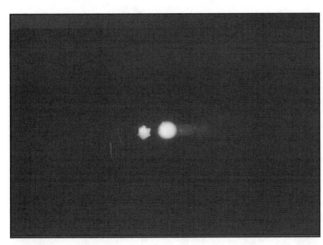

Figure 4-5B. Example of pinpoint illumination (anterior chamber). (Photo by Val Sanders.)

Pinpoint (Conical Section)

Pinpoint illumination is used to detect suspended particles in a liquid (in the eye, the aqueous) or gas. The principle is the same as a beam of sunlight streaming through a room, illuminating airborne dust particles. This occurrence is known as Tyndall's phenomenon. Lower the height of the beam to form a single round beam of light. Increase the intensity of your light source to the highest setting. Direct the beam so that it enters the cornea temporal to the pupil and strikes the iris nasal to the pupil (Figures 4-5A and 4-5B). Increase magnification to 16X or 25X. Focus in the anterior chamber between the lens and corneal endothelium. Continue to make slight focusing movements in and out in order to sweep the entire chamber. If the eye is inflamed, cells (immune cells) and flare (or ray, clumps of protein) may be present in the aqueous. Locating the cells may be facilitated if you gently oscillate the illuminator. Pinpoint illumination is easier if the pupil is not dilated.

Observe: cells, flare

Figure 4-6A. Schematic of specular reflection. (Adapted and reprinted with permission from *Ophthalmic Photography*, SLACK Incorporated.)

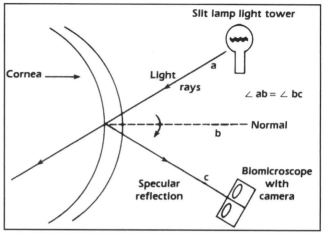

Figure 4-6B. Example of specular reflection. (Photo by Val Sanders.)

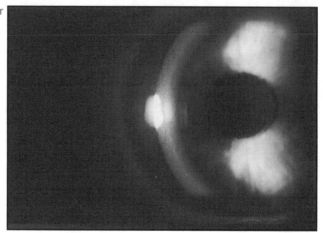

Specular Reflection

Specular reflection is used to visualize the integrity of the corneal and lens surfaces. If the surface is smooth, the reflection will be smooth and regular; if the surface is broken or rough, the reflection will likewise be irregular or appear to be textured. Its most common use is in evaluating the general appearance of the corneal endothelium. In this technique, position the illuminator about 30 degrees to one side and the microscope 30 degrees to the other side. The angle of the illuminator to the microscope must be equal and opposite (Figures 4-6A and 4-6B).

To visualize the endothelium, start with lower magnification (10X to 16X). Direct a relatively narrow beam onto the cornea so that the reflection of light off of the epithelium dazzles you. Then move the light a little to the side, and look adjacent to it, at the reflection from the endothelial surface. Now switch to the highest magnification available. Lowering the height of the slit beam may reduce glare. Widening the slit will increase the field but decrease contrast. The endothelium is best viewed using only one ocular, so you may want to close one eye. This technique is difficult to master, partly because the cells have such low contrast, and takes some experimentation and experience. Cell counts done strictly by slit lamp observation are not generally accepted. Contact specular microscopy is much more accurate.

Observe: corneal epithelium and endothelium, endothelial mosaic, lens surfaces

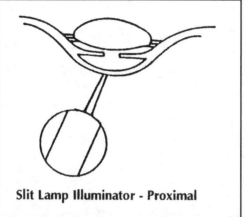

Slit Lamp Illuminator - Proximal

Figure 4-7A. Schematic of proximal illumination. (Adapted with permission from *Ophthalmic Photography*, SLACK Incorporated.)

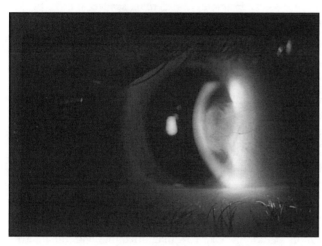

Figure 4-7B. Example of proximal illumination. (Photo by Val Sanders.)

Indirect Illumination

Indirect illumination provides more detail than diffuse or direct illumination. In these methods, abnormalities are not illuminated by shining the slit beam directly on them. Rather they are lit up by light that is reflected off of an uninvolved area. The microscope itself is focused at a different depth or plane than the light source.

Proximal

This illumination technique is used to observe internal detail, depth, and density. Use a short, fairly narrow slit beam. Place the beam at the border of the structure or pathology (Figures 4-7A and 4-7B). The light will be scattered into the surrounding tissue, creating a light background that highlights the edges of the abnormality. Depending on the density of the abnormality, the light from behind may reflect through, allowing detailed examination of the internal structure of the pathology.

Observe: corneal opacities (edema, infiltrates, vessels, foreign bodies), lens, iris

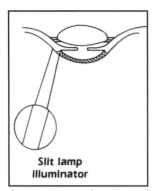

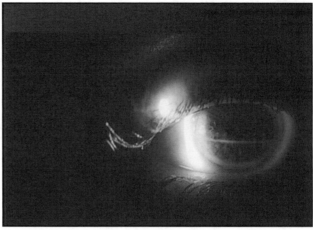

Figure 4-8A. Schematic of sclerotic scatter. (Reprinted with permission from *Ophthalmic Photography*, SLACK Incorporated.)

Figure 4-8B. Example of sclerotic scatter. (Photo by Val Sanders.)

Sclerotic Scatter

This method is useful to view the distribution of corneal pathology, making it especially useful in contact lens evaluation (see Chapter 9). A tall, wide beam is directed onto the limbal area. The illuminator should be slightly offset for this technique and directed from a moderate angle. (The illuminator is almost always left in a straight-ahead position. In a horizontal prism reflected microscope, the illuminator is offset by simply rotating the slit scanning control ring. If your slit lamp has a vertical illumination source, turn the slit centering knob near the bottom of the illumination arm.) When the light is properly aligned with regard to the eye, a ring of light will appear around the cornea. The light is absorbed and scattered through the cornea (see Figures 4-8A and 4-8B), highlighting pathology. Use 10X magnification, with the microscope directed straight ahead. This technique is easiest if the patient is not dilated so that the iris provides a contrasting dark background.

Observe: general pattern of corneal opacities

Retroillumination

Retroillumination is used to evaluate the optical qualities of a structure. The light strikes the object of interest from a point behind the object and is then reflected back to the observer. Thus, it is similar to a silhouette. Some professionals advocate setting the slit beam slightly off center (via the slit scanning control ring or the slit centering knob) for these techniques. The authors prefer to leave the slit beam in its usual position.

Direct Retroillumination From the Iris

This illumination method is used to view corneal pathology. A moderately wide slit beam is aimed toward the iris directly behind the corneal abnormality (Figures 4-9A and 4-9B). Use a magnification of 16X to 25X, and direct the light from 45 degrees. The microscope is directed straight ahead. The light strikes the iris, highlighting the corneal pathology on which you focus the microscope. The beam of light must pass behind rather than striking on the pathology for this

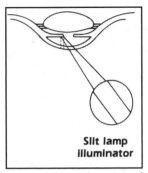

Figure 4-9A. Schematic of direct retroillumination from the iris. (Reprinted with permission from *Ophthalmic Photography*, SLACK Incorporated.)

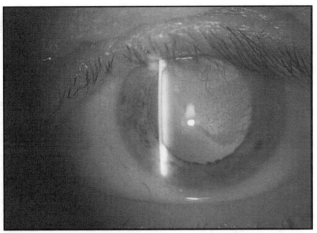

Figure 4-9B. Example of direct retroillumination from the iris. (Photo by Val Sanders.)

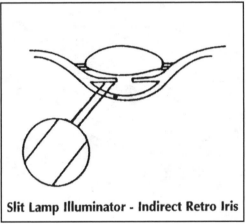

Figure 4-10A. Schematic of indirect retroillumination from the iris. Note that the corneal pathology to be viewed is not directly in the beam. (Adapted with permission from *Ophthalmic Photography*, SLACK Incorporated.)

technique to be effective. Vary the beam angle slightly until you get the best detail. This technique is best accomplished if the patient is not dilated.

Observe: cornea

Indirect Retroillumination From the Iris

The technique is performed as with direct retroillumination (above), but the beam is directed to an area of the iris bordering the portion of the iris behind the pathology (Figures 4-10A and 4-10B). This provides a dark background, allowing corneal opacities to be viewed with more contrast.

The angles are also evaluated with this technique. (The reason that chamber depth/angle evaluation is an indirect method is that you are not looking at the cornea or the iris, but at the dark interval next to the beam.) See Chapter 3 for details on examining the chamber and angles.

Observe: cornea, angles

Figure 4-10B. Example of indirect iris retroillumination (angle). (Photo by Val Sanders.)

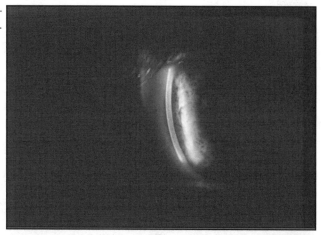

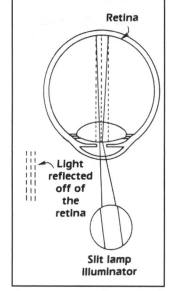

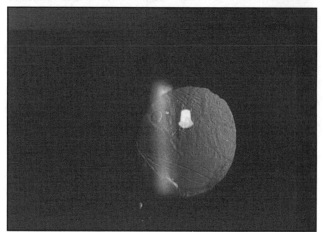

Figure 4-11A. Schematic of retroillumination from the retina. (Reprinted with permission from *Ophthalmic Photography*, SLACK Incorporated.)

Figure 4-11B. Example of retroillumination from the retina. (Photo by Val Sanders.)

Retroillumination From the Fundus (Red Reflex)

In this technique, you are seeking to visualize media clarity and opacities. The light is directed so that it strikes the fundus and creates a *glow* behind the abnormality (Figures 4-11A and 4-11B). The defect creates a shadow in the light. Use a moderate beam projected through a dilated pupil. The slit beam and microscope must be nearly coaxial; direct the illumination proximally at 2 to 4 degrees. Shorten the beam to the height of the pupil to avoid reflecting the bright light off of the iris. If your instrument has the capability to do so, you might also adjust the beam into a crescent so its shape will fit the pupil. (Check your user's manual.) Focus the microscope directly on the pathology using 10X to 16X magnification. Opacities will appear in silhouette. This view is best accomplished if the pupil is dilated.

Observe: cornea, lens, vitreous

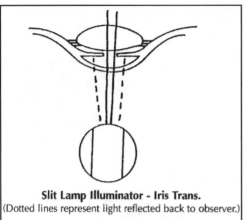

Slit Lamp Illuminator - Iris Trans.
(Dotted lines represent light reflected back to observer.)

Figure 4-12A. Schematic of iris transillumination. (Adapted with permission from *Ophthalmic Photography*, SLACK Incorporated.)

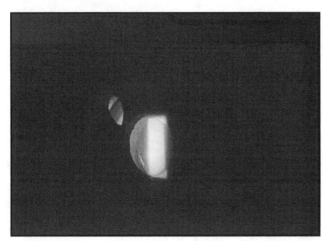

Figure 4-12B. Example of iris transillumination. (Photo by Val Sanders.)

Transillumination

In transillumination, a structure (in the eye, the iris) is evaluated by how light passes through it.

Iris Transillumination

This technique also takes advantage of the red reflex. The pupil must be at mid mydriasis (3 to 4 mm when light stimulated). Place the light source coaxial (directly in line) with the microscope. Use a full circle beam of light equal to the size of the pupil. Project the light through the pupil and into the eye (Figures 4-12A and 4-12B). If the light falls on the iris at all, your view will be diminished. Focus the microscope on the iris. Magnification of 10X to 16X is adequate. *Observe: iris defects (they will glow with the orange light reflected from the fundus)*

Illumination Mnemonic

To help you remember which illumination technique falls under which heading, the authors have developed the following mnemonic:

1. **Diffuse**
2. **Direct**

Beam	Beagles
Tangential	Take
Pinpoint	Pills
Specular Reflection	Sparingly

3. **Indirect**

Proximal	Precise
Sclerotic Scatter	Scientists
Retroillumination	Receive
Transillumination	Training

Chapter 5

Slit Lamp Findings

KEY POINTS

- It is usually best to record findings rather than diagnoses.

- The system of grading certain findings is subjective, or relative to the opinion of the observer.

- Measuring the size of a lesion at the slit lamp may be accomplished with an external ruler, a measuring grid in the ocular, or the slit beam itself.

- Drawing with colored pencils as a code can be a very useful tool in documentation of certain structures or findings.

Chapters 2 through 4 have detailed the methods used in examining the eye with the slit lamp microscope. This chapter is a list of common slit lamp findings, describing the appearance of the abnormality along with pertinent documentation instructions (given as Documentation). The notes on documentation are a variety of suggestions; it may not be necessary to complete each one. The word *note* means merely to note in the chart that the finding exists. Remember that it is sometimes pertinent to document the *absence* of particular findings to indicate that the structure in question was indeed examined for a particular entity. It is also worth noting that the record of the slit lamp exam should usually give findings, not diagnoses. For example, it would be incorrect to write "2+ blepharitis" as the slit lamp entry. Instead, the observer should notate the findings themselves, such as "2+ lid edema and erythema, 1+ lash loss, 3+ crusting." Having said that, we admit that we have included some diagnoses in the listings. You and/or your supervisor should decide how to document slit lamp findings and diagnoses in your particular office or clinic.

We have alphabetized the findings given in each list. It is probably best to read through the listing once or twice before attempting to use it in the exam room. This is because, while you may look for the word "redness," we may have chosen to list the finding as *erythema* or *injection.* Other terms fall into the same problem category. If you scan through the lists a time or two, you will be able to pick out the appropriate findings when you need them. Some of the more common diagnoses (such as blepharitis, dry eye, iritis, etc) are listed in Chapter 6. (Check the index if what you are looking for is not listed as a finding.)

Criteria for several certification exams include "common ocular disorders" without being any more specific than that. Candidates for these exams should probably familiarize themselves with most of the findings listed. Icons appear beside items that are specifically mentioned or implied as exam criteria.

The Subjective Grading System

An important but confusing part of documenting abnormalities is the subjective grading system. Even the term "subjective" causes confusion because such grading occurs during the objective examination. Some clarification seems to be in order.

First, many of the patient's symptoms are subjective. These are symptoms that the patient tells us about but that we cannot see, such as pain. Other findings are objective, which do not involve the patient's ability to report them. We can see them ourselves when we examine the patient. Cell and flare in the anterior chamber is an objective finding; the patient does not (and cannot) tell us about it, but we can see it. Other findings fall into both realms. The patient may say, "My right eye is red," which is subjective. Through the slit lamp, we can also see the injection whether the patient has reported it or not, which is objective. The slit lamp exam is an objective test.

Grading pathology and other findings, although they are discovered during the objective examination, is subjective on the part of the examiner. Here, subjective means that the assignment of a rating to a finding is dependent on the observer's opinion. You may look at the patient and grade her lid edema as 2+. Another clinician may rate the same finding (same patient, same day, same time) as 1+ or 3+. The best we can advise you is that if you are auxiliary personnel, try to learn the grading system of your employer. As you examine more and more eyes, you will get a feel for how marked a finding is. If you are a physician, do your best to teach your grading philosophy to your staff.

With that said, we would like to offer our own opinion about how to grade your findings. Some prefer a numbered grading system. If you use this, then 0 means that a finding is absent. 1+ would indicate that a finding is just barely perceptible. A full-blown case would be referred to as 4+. Using this schematic, 2+ and 3+ would fall somewhere in between. This system is sometimes complicated by interjecting half steps in between, such as 2.5+. You can decide whether this practice is truly necessary or not.

The plus sign itself can be a point of contention. To some, the "+" is used to indicate a half step. In this book, we are generally avoiding half steps.

Instead of numbers, specific terms can be used, including "none, absent, bare trace, trace, slight, moderate, marked, severe" and other such words. This is even more subjective than the numbering system. If everyone uses a scale of 0+ to 4+, then we have a better chance of understanding what 2+ means. Who is to say what the difference really is between *bare trace* and *trace*? The dilemma of subjective grading is not likely to be solved.

Measuring

Measuring the size of a finding can be an important part of the slit lamp examination. A record of a lesion's size from one exam to the next allows us to monitor for growth or resolution. Obviously, a lesion may be measured using a hand held ruler with one hand while observing through the slit lamp. Admittedly, this is awkward. It is far easier to use an ocular that has a ruler built in to the reticule. A third method is possible with vertical illumination source models. First, the slit is rotated to coincide with the axis that you want to measure. Then, the slit beam height is reduced or lengthened to match the lesion. The measurement is read from a slit length display window on the illumination arm. Prior to using this method, the beam should be calibrated against a millimeter rule.

External Findings (Lids/Lacrimal)

- **blepharospasm** – lid twitch.

Doc: note

- **bruising** (hematoma) – common after lid surgery or injury.

Doc: note, grade 1+ to 4+, give location, draw

- **burn** – injury caused by heat.

Doc: note, give location, estimate percentage of dermis that is burned, estimate degree (first degree, skin red and usually moist; second degree, blistering; third degree, full thickness, may be charred, lashes and hair pull out easily), draw

- **collarettes** – blepharitis/granulated eyelids. Little white greasy crusty flakes surrounding the base of the lashes.

Doc: note, grade 1+ to 4+

- **coloboma** – a vertical fissure in the lid where the tissues did not fuse during embryonic development.

Doc: note

- **crusting/matting** – lashes are glued together with dried matter.

Doc: note, grade 1+ to 4+

- **distichia** – extra row of lashes often growing from the openings of the meibomian glands.

Doc: note, give location if appropriate

- **ectropion** – lower lid sags out, exposing conjunctiva.

Doc: note, grade 1+ to 4+ (1+ is barely turned out, 4+ looks like a Basset hound)

- **edema** – swelling.

Doc: note, give location, grade 1+ to 4+ (4+ is swollen shut)

- **entropion** – lower lid flips in with lashes rubbing cornea.

Doc: note, grade 1+ to 4+

- **erythema** – redness.

Doc: note, grade 1+ to 4+ (1+ is barely pink, 4+ is fire engine red)

- **froth** – tiny white bubbles at lower lid or in corner of eye, an indication of overactive meibomian glands.

Doc: note, grade 1+ to 4+

- **laceration** – cut.

Doc: note, give location, measure, draw, note other lid structures involved (such as punctum)

- **lash loss** – fewer lashes than normal, usually due to chronic infection or habit of picking lashes out.

Doc: note, give location, grade 1+ to 4+

- **lesion** (Table 5-1) – general term for any growth on the lids/brows. Could include skin tag, cyst, mole (nevus), wart, etc.

Doc: note, location, measure, describe (crusty, cratered center, brown, flat, etc), draw

- **lid closure** – whether or not the upper lid comes all the way down to the lower lid when patient blinks or closes eye. If upper meets lower, closure is "complete." If there is a gap and some of the eyeball (usually the cornea) is not covered, this is termed "incomplete."

Doc: note if complete or incomplete. If incomplete, give exposed area of globe in fractions (ie, "lower third")

- **lid lag** – the upper lid does not immediately follow the eye when the patient looks down (Von Graefe's sign).

Doc: note

- **lid position** – location of the upper and lower lid margins when the eye is opened. May include ectropion, entropion, inferior scleral show (exposure), failure of lower punctum to contact globe, ptosis.

Doc: note, describe, measure fissure openings (if ptosis)

- **lid retraction** – the upper lid margin is above or the lower lid margin is below normal when the eye is opened. This may be marked enough to produce scleral show.

Doc: note, describe

- **notching** (Figure 5-2) – a nick in the lid margin often associated with trauma, surgery, or chronic blepharitis.

Doc: note, give location, draw

- **packed meibomian glands** (meibomian plugs) – looks like little droplets or whitish "plugs" along the lower lid. This is oil at the opening of the glands.

Doc: note

TABLE 5-1
Common Lid Lesions

- **Basal cell carcinoma** (Figure 5-1)**:** depression in center, white border, small vessels, may be scaly, may bleed.

- **Chalazion:** swollen meibomian gland in lid. If you pull the lid back, you can see it from the bulbar conjunctival side, too. Usually a round smooth nodule under skin. May have a *head* on it. If head is visible on lid, it is termed "pointing to the skin." If head is on conjunctival side (the more common case), it is said to be "pointing to the conjunctiva." Early chalazion may have more generalized swelling with the knot only slightly evident.

- **Cyst:** fluid-filled vesicle.

- **Hemangioma:** a congenital vascular tumor that may vary in color from bright red to blue to violet.

- **Hordeola:** sty; inflamed oil gland at base of lash follicle; tender red lump at lid margin.

- **Kaposi's sarcoma:** a reddish-blue nodule associated with autoimmune disease (AIDS).

- **Melanoma:** may have jagged or uneven edges; may start near a mole; may be colorless; may turn brown, tan, or black; may have blue or red sections.

- **Milia:** tiny, elevated, singular white nodules (may occur in groups).

- **Mole (nevus):** usually present at birth, may be pigmented or flesh-toned, symmetrical.

- **Molluscum contagiosum:** small, waxy, wartlike lesion often with a "dip" in the center; usually found on lid margin.

- **Seborrheic keratoses (senile verruca):** appear in older individuals; flat, bumpy surface, often pigmented.

- **Skin tag (cutaneous horn):** cylindrical, flesh-colored outgrowth.

- **Squamous cell carcinoma:** may start as nodules or red patches; later looks like a wart, erodes and ulcerates.

- **Wart (verruca):** elevated, with a bumpy surface.

- **Xanthelasma:** yellow, dull, fairly flat deposits usually on the upper lids, may be on lower lids.

Figure 5-1. Basal cell carcinoma of the lower lid. (Photo by Val Sanders.)

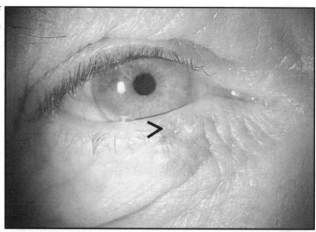

Figure 5-2. Lid notching. (Photo by Val Sanders.)

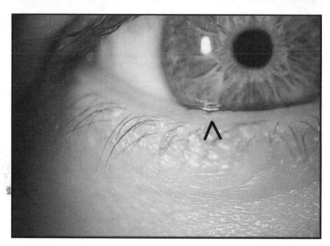

- **port wine stain** – a congenital, flat, red area (looks like the skin was stained).

Doc: note, describe, location, draw, measure

- **ptosis** – lid droop.

Doc: note, measure fissure opening (this may be done with a measuring reticule in the slit lamp ocular), draw

- **reflux** – purulent material that is regurgitated out of the lower punctum when you press on the nasolacrimal area.

Doc: note as positive (present) or negative (absent)

- **trichiasis** – in-turned lash(es), may rub on the cornea.

Doc: note, location, number, draw

The Globe

Tears

- **break up time (BUT)** – see Chapter 3.

Doc: note time to break-up

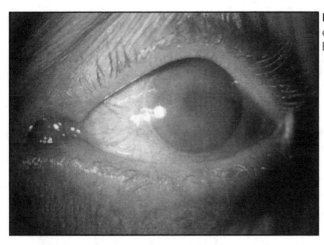

Figure 5-3. Ciliary flush with corneal edema (note haze). (Photo by Val Sanders.)

- **debris** – foreign matter in tear film.

Doc: note, identify source if possible (ie, mascara, ointment, etc), grade 1+ to 4+

- **discharge** – abnormal excretion.

Doc: note, describe (purulent, mucopurulent, serous), grade 1+ to 4+ or use words (scanty, profuse, etc)

- **epiphora** – excess tearing.

Doc: note

- **matter** – purulent discharge.

Doc: note, describe (stringy, yellow, etc), grade 1+ to 4+ or use words (scanty, profuse, etc)

- **oily** – a sheen of oil can be seen on the surface of the tear film.

Doc: note, grade 1+ to 4+

Conjunctiva, Episclera, Sclera

- **ciliary flush** (limbal injection, Figure 5-3) – injection of the deep vessels around the limbus. These vessels do not move when pushed with a cotton-tipped applicator, nor do they bleach with phenylephrine.

Doc: note, grade 1+ to 4+

- **color** – the white of the eye should be white, but may be yellow in the elderly or jaundiced and bluish in children or patients with keratoconus or high myopia.

Doc: note, describe

- **conjunctival cyst** – looks like a little fluid-filled translucent blister on the conjunctiva.

Doc: note, measure, draw, give location

- **dryness** – if the conjunctiva is dry, you will see it being dragged by the upper lid during the blink.

Doc: note

- **edema (chemosis)** – swelling of the conjunctiva, looks like there is "too much" conjunctiva, that it is overflowing.

Doc: note, grade 1+ to 4+ (1+ is just noticeable, like a tiny extra fold of conjunctiva. 4+ looks like a lot of fluid behind the conjunctiva, making it bulge out past the cornea.)

- **follicles** – smooth yellow/clear bumps on palpebral conjunctiva. Sign of viral infection. In contrast to papillae, follicles do not have central blood vessels.

Doc: note, grade 1+ to 4+

Figure 5-4. Mild conjunctival injection; note blood vessels to right of cornea. (Photo by Val Sanders.)

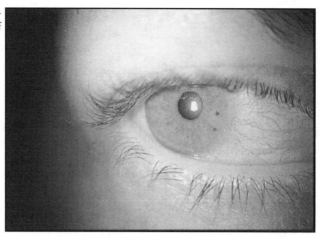

TABLE 5-2
Grading Injection*

Feature	Grade
No injection present	0
Slight limbal (mild segmented), bulbar (mild regional), and/or palpebral injection	1+
Mild limbal (mild circumcorneal), bulbar (mild diffuse), and/or palpebral injection	2+
Significant limbal (marked segmented), bulbar (marked regional or diffuse), or palpebral injection	3+
Severe limbal (marked circum-corneal), bulbar (diffuse episcleral or scleral), or palpebral injection	4+

*Adapted from FDA document *Premarket Notification Guidance Document for Daily Wear Contact Lenses.*

- **foreign body** – anything that does not naturally belong in or on the conjunctiva. (The most interesting conjunctival foreign body I have ever seen was an ant. The insect had bitten into the conjunctiva before it died. The doctor had to numb the eye and cut the ant out!)

Doc: note, identify (if possible), give location, draw

- **injection** (hyperemia; Figure 5-4) – general redness of conjunctiva. If injection is mainly around limbus and not generalized, it is described as "limbal injection."

Doc: graded 1+ to 4+ (1+ is just noticeably pink, 4+ is glow-in-the-dark) (Table 5-2)

- **laceration** – cut.

Doc: note, measure, draw, give location

- **leash vessel(s)** (Figure 5-5) – a prominent red blood vessel (conjunctiva is not totally injected). If the vessel is in the conjunctiva or surface episclera, it will bleach with topical phenylephrine. Deeper episcleral or scleral vessels will not bleach.

Doc: note location (directional or by the clock), draw

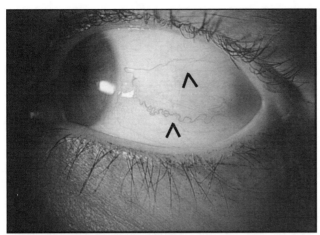

Figure 5-5. Conjunctival leash vessels. (Photo by Val Sanders.)

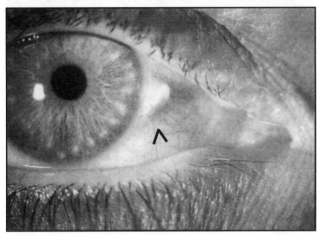

Figure 5-6. Pinguecula. (Photo by Val Sanders.)

- **papillae** – little elevated lesions on palpebral conjunctiva that have blood vessels in the center. Sign of infection or allergy.

Doc: note, grade 1+ to 4+

- **pinguecula** (Figure 5-6) – yellow or white roundish growth at the limbus nasally or temporally.

Doc: note, give location by the clock, may draw and measure

- **prolapsed tear gland** – a yellowish mass visible under conjunctiva of the upper lid.

Doc: note

- **scleral show** – the lid does not cover the eye up to the cornea; some of the sclera is exposed.

Doc: note, describe (inferior, superior), measure, draw

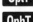

- **scleral thinning** – bluish areas where the sclera has thinned to the point that the black choroid shows underneath (but has not broken through).

Doc: note, give location, draw

- **subconjunctival hemorrhage** (SCH; Figure 5-7A) – blood-red patch on the sclera, under the conjunctiva; analogous to a bruise elsewhere on the body.

Doc: note, give location, draw

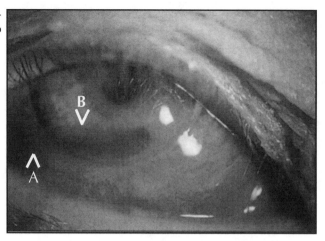

Figure 5-7. Subconjunctival hemorrhage (A) with Hyphema (B). (Photo by Val Sanders.)

- **uveal prolapse** – a portion of the uvea protrudes through the sclera; the uvea is black and easily visible against the white sclera.

Doc: note, give location, draw

Cornea

Documentation by Drawings

A system of documenting corneal pathology by hand-drawn illustrations has been described by several authors. Waring and Laibson suggest the following color scheme:

- black
    - solid line – sutures
    - dotted line – contact lens
    - dots – guttata
- blue: edema
    - wavy lines – Descemet's folds
    - tiny circles – epithelial edema
- brown: pigment, iris
- red: blood, rose bengal
    - thin solid line – superficial vessels
    - thick solid line – stromal vessels
    - dotted line – ghost vessels
- green: fluorescein, lens, vitreous
    - solid wavy lines – filaments
- yellow: infiltrate, hypopyon, keratitic precipitates

In addition, the location of corneal findings may be designated by a system described by Josephson and Caffery. Zone 1 is the central 6.00 mm of the cornea. The peripheral cornea is divided into four zones by lines at 1:30, 4:30, 7:30, and 10:30. The superior section is Zone 2, and the numbers continue clockwise so that the section on the examiner's right is Zone 3, inferior is Zone 4, and Zone 5 is on the examiner's left.

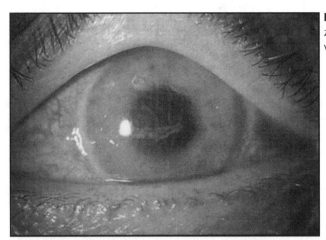

Figure 5-8. Corneal abrasion (horizontal stained area) with striae (faint vertical lines). (Photo by Val Sanders.)

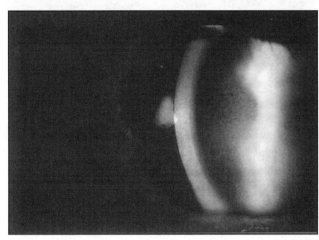

Figure 5-9. Corneal dystrophy. (Photo by Val Sanders.)

Findings

- **abrasion** (Figure 5-8) – scratch. Stains with fluorescein.

Doc: note give location, measure or estimate size, draw

- **arcus senilis** – white-gray ring just inside the limbus, may or may not extend 360 degrees.

Doc: note, draw

- **band keratopathy** – a white band of calcification that extends across the center of the cornea to the limbus at 3:00 and 9:00. There may be clear gaps, giving it the appearance of Swiss cheese.

Doc: note, grade 1+ to 4+, draw

- **corneal diameter** – can be measured with reticule in ocular; average is 11.00 to 12.00 mm.

Doc: measure

- **dellen** – depression in the corneal surface next to the limbus. Fluorescein may pool in it, but it does not stain. May occur after muscle, pterygium, or filtration surgery.

Doc: note, draw, measure, give location

- **dystrophy** (Figure 5-9) – grainy textured appearance on back surface of cornea. May look like a fingerprint on a piece of tape. May have a ground-glass, glittering appearance or an opaque pattern (through which endothelium may not be visible).

Doc: note, grade 1+ to 4+

TABLE 5-3
Grading Corneal Haze*

Feature	Grade
Clear	0
Between clear and trace; barely perceptible	0.5+
Trace; easily seen with slit lamp	1+
Mild haze	2+
Moderate haze, pronounced, iris details still visible, AC reaction not visible	3+
Marked haze, scarring, iris details obscured	4+

*Adapted with permission from Stein HA, Cheskes AT, Stein RM. *The Excimer: Fundamentals and Clinical Use.* Thorofare, NJ: SLACK Incorporated; 1995.

- **edema** (see Figure 5-3) – using a narrow beam, the corneal section looks larger/thicker than usual. The surface may appear to have bubbles or folds. Cornea may look cloudy.

Doc: note, describe location (epithelial or stromal), grade (Table 5-3), draw

- **filaments** – tiny spiral strands that are attached at one end to the corneal epithelium. They stain with fluorescein or rose bengal.

Doc: note, give location, estimate number, draw

- **Fleischer ring** – an epithelial iron ring that is incident with the base of the corneal cone in keratoconus; best viewed with red-free filter.

Doc: note, draw

- **foreign body** – anything that does not naturally belong on/in the cornea.

Doc: note, identify (if possible), give location, draw

- **ghost vessels** – abnormal corneal vessels that have subsided (ie, are no longer filled with blood).

Doc: note, give location by the clock, draw

- **guttata** (Figure 5-10) – tiny brown dots on back surface of cornea, generally concentrated centrally and in a uniform pattern. Appear as holes when using specular reflection.

Doc: note, grade 1+ to 4+

- **Hudson-Stahli line** – a thin, black, horizontal iron line on the corneal epithelium at the approximate place where the upper and lower lids meet when the eye is closed; nicely viewed with red-free filter.

Doc: note, draw

- **infiltrates** (Figure 5-11) – whitish "cloud" within the corneal tissue, under the epithelium, often surrounding an ulcer or foreign body. They are actually white blood cells that have entered the cornea to fight infection. If they do not stain, they are not infections and thus termed "sterile." If there is stain, then they are associated with infection.

Doc: note, draw

- **iron lines** – thin black line(s) on the corneal epithelium. Nicely viewed with red-free filter.

Doc: note, give location, draw

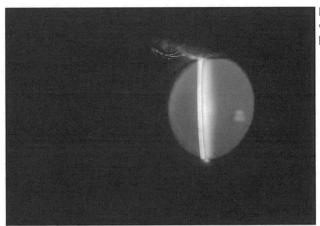

Figure 5-10. Corneal guttata as viewed with fundus retroillumination. (Photo by Val Sanders.)

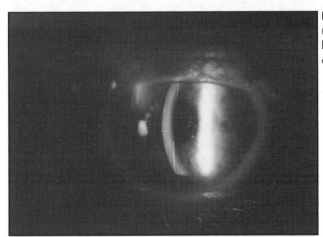

Figure 5-11. Subepithelial infiltrates (to right of beam on cornea, left of beam on iris) seen in epidemic kerato-conjunctivitis. (Photo by Val Sanders.)

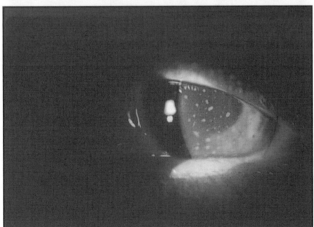

Figure 5-12. Keratitic precipitates. (Photo by Val Sanders.)

- **keratitic precipitates** (KP's; Figure 5-12) – white-yellow roundish glossy blobs (dubbed "mutton fat" because of their appearance) or a fine "dusting" of white precipitates. Appear in a random pattern (as opposed to guttata) on back surface of cornea, usually on the inferior one-third. Larger and whiter than guttata. Often present in iritis and uveitis and are a

Figure 5-13. Krukenberg spindles (faintly visible to right of beam on cornea). (Photo by Val Sanders.)

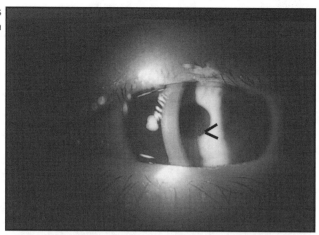

Figure 5-14. Corneal pannus. (Photo by Val Sanders.)

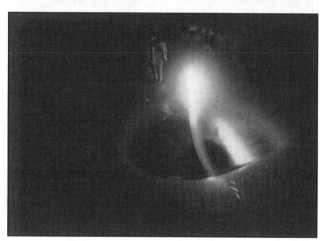

sign of inflammation. Often go away when inflammation clears up. Some may linger, and therefore look browner and not as glossy.

Doc: note, grade 1+ to 4+ (according to how many and how much of the cornea is covered)

- **Krukenberg spindles** (Figure 5-13) – these are tiny brown dots lined up vertically over the central cornea (on its back surface). May look like a dusting of spatter-paint on the endothelium, broader at its base.

Doc: note, grade 1+ to 4+

- **opacity** – cloudy or opaque area.

Doc: note, describe, give location, draw

- **pannus** (Figure 5-14) – fibrous area with blood vessels that extends from the limbus onto the cornea.

Doc: note, give location, draw

- **phlyctenule** – white limbal elevation with blood vessels on the conjunctival side.

Doc: note, give location, draw

- **pterygium** (Figure 5-15) – wedge of flesh extending from conjunctiva onto external cornea. Usually nasal, may be temporal.

Doc: note, give location, measure, draw

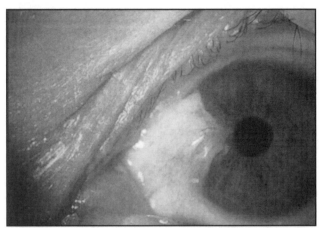

Figure 5-15. Pterygium. (Photo by Val Sanders.)

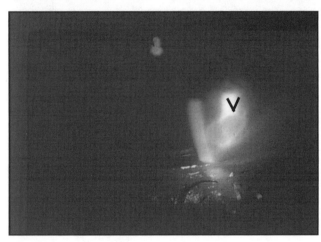

Figure 5-16. Corneal ulcer. (Photo by Val Sanders.)

- **rust ring** – rust stain on epithelium (may be lower layers as well) surrounding a metallic foreign body or remaining after removal of a metallic foreign body.

Doc: note, measure, give location, draw

- **scar** – an opacity caused by injury to corneal layers below the epithelium.

Doc: note, measure, give location, draw

- **striae** (See Figure 5-8) – these are wrinkles on the back surface of the cornea. Common after surgery, not seen if IOP is high (pressure presses them out).

Doc: note, grade 1+ to 4+

- **ulcer** (Figure 5-16) – appears as round, whitish, hazy area. Stains with fluorescein. May be surrounded by white blood cells in the stroma (infiltrates).

Doc: note, give location, measure, draw, note presence of infiltrates and/or discharge

- **vascularization** (neovascularization; Figure 5-17) – growth of abnormal blood vessels into/onto cornea. There are normal vessels at the limbus; usually these loop back into the conjunctiva. Abnormal vessels usually branch (do not loop) and extend further out into the cornea than the normal vessels.

Doc: note, give location by the clock, draw, grade (Table 5-4)

Figure 5-17. Corneal vascularization (note faint vessels on superior cornea). (Photo by Val Sanders.)

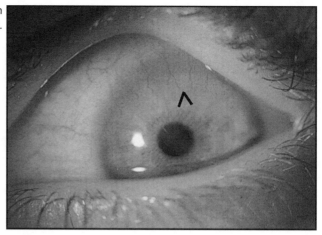

TABLE 5-4
Grading Corneal Vascularization*

Feature	Grade
No vascular changes	0
Congestion and dilation of the limbal vessels; single vessel extension <1.5 mm	1+
Extension of multiple vessels <1.5 mm	2+
Extension of multiple limbal vessels 1.5 mm to 2.5 mm	3+
Segmented or circumscribed extension of limbal vessels >2.5 mm or to within 3.0 mm of corneal apex	4+

*Adapted from FDA document *Premarket Notification Guidance Document for Daily Wear Contact Lenses*.

Corneal Staining (Figure 5-18, Table 5-5)

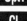

- **abrasion** – injured area that stains, may be fine linear scratches or large area with irregular-shaped borders.

Doc: note, describe, location, draw

- **bullae** – blisterlike bubbles on cornea. If they stain, they have broken through.

Doc: note, location, draw

- **dendrite** (Figure 5-19) – tree-branch area of staining typical of Herpes simplex.

Doc: note, draw

- **dry spots** (Figure 5-20) – larger stained areas, usually have smooth edges, may be one or several. Use rose bengal or fluorescein.

Doc: note, location, number, draw

- **punctate epithelial erosion (PEE) or superficial punctate keratopathy (SPK)** (Figure 5-21) – tiny dots of stain. May look like spatter paint.

Doc: note, give location (inferior, interpalpebral, superior), describe pattern (localized, scattered, diffuse), comment on number (do not count, just write "few," "dense," etc), grade 1+ to 4+

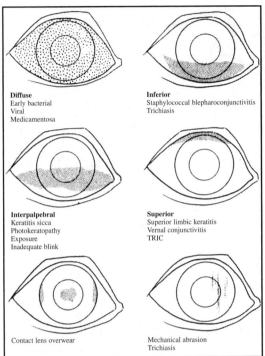

Diffuse
Early bacterial
Viral
Medicamentosa

Inferior
Staphylococcal blepharoconjunctivitis
Trichiasis

Interpalpebral
Keratitis sicca
Photokeratopathy
Exposure
Inadequate blink

Superior
Superior limbic keratitis
Vernal conjunctivitis
TRIC

Contact lens overwear

Mechanical abrasion
Trichiasis

Figure 5-18. Staining patterns of the cornea and conjunctiva in various disease states. TRIC = trachoma-inclusion conjunctivitis (group). (Reprinted with permission from Langston D, ed. *Manual of Ocular Diagnosis and Therapy*. 2nd ed. Little, Brown and Co/Lippincott-Raven.)

TABLE 5-5
Grading Corneal Staining*

Feature	Grade
No staining	0
Minimal superficial staining or stippling	1+
Regional or diffuse punctate staining	2+
Significant dense coalesced staining, corneal abrasion, or foreign body tracks	3+
Severe abrasions >2.00 mm diameter, ulcerations, epithelial loss, or full thickness abrasion	4+

*Adapted from FDA document *Premarket Notification Guidance Document for Daily Wear Contact Lenses*.

Figure 5-19. Herpetic dendrite. (Photo by Val Sanders.)

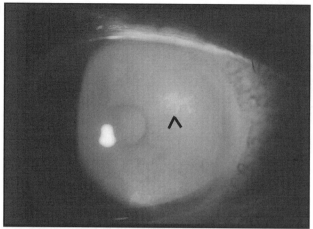

Figure 5-20. Dry eye stained with rose bengal (lower left quadrant). (Photo by Val Sanders.)

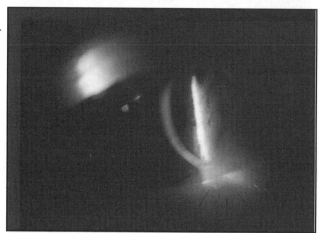

Figure 5-21. Superficial punctate keratopathy (lower left quadrant). (Photo by Val Sanders.)

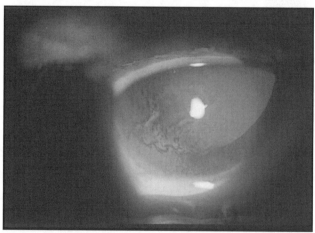

TABLE 5-6
Grading Angles

Features	Grade
Closed angle	0
Angle extremely narrow, probable closure	1+
Angle moderately narrow, possible closure	2+
Angle moderately open, closure not possible	3+
Angle wide open, closure not possible	4+

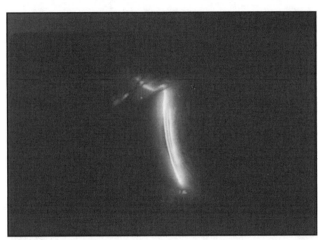

Figure 5-22. Narrow angle (note lack of shadow interval). (Photo by Val Sanders.)

- **stained area** – good junk term for corneal staining that you cannot identify.

Doc: note, location, comment on pattern, draw

- **tear film** – the tear film (with fluorescein) should spread smoothly over the cornea with each blink, not bead up as on a freshly-waxed car. (See Chapter 3 on break up time.)

Doc: note if decreased BUT

- **ulcer** (See Figure 5-16) – usually a roundish area of staining associated with infection (virus, bacteria, or fungus). May be surrounded by infiltrates.

Doc: note, give location, measure, draw, note presence of infiltrates and/or discharge

Note: corneal staining related to contact lens wear is discussed in Chapter 9.

Anterior Chamber and Angles

- **angle opening**- see Chapter 3.

Doc: graded 1+ to 4+ (Table 5-6) or merely termed "open," "narrow" (Figure 5-22), or "closed"

- **cell(s)** – blood cells floating free (circulating, actually) in the aqueous. They are associated with inflammation and are commonly seen after surgery or trauma. They are very tiny and look like dust particles in the sunlight. These are moving targets!

Doc: note; grade 1+ to 4+ (Table 5-7); also may describe, such as "trace" or even "single cell"

TABLE 5-7
Grading Cell (1.00 mm Conical Beam)

Cell #	Grade
1 to 10	Trace
10 to 20	1+
20 to 30	2+
30 to 40	3+
40 up to hypopyon	4+

Figure 5-23. Flat anterior chamber (note curvature of the iris behind cornea). (Photo by Val Sanders.)

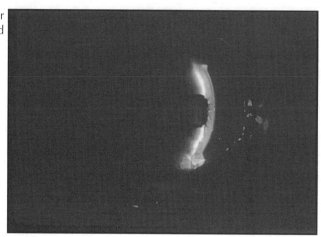

OphA

- **depth** – the distance from the back of the cornea to the front of the iris. Myopes are usually deep, hyperopes may be shallower. Anterior chamber (A/C) is said to be flat if iris bows forward against the cornea (Figure 5-23). Flat chamber usually occurs after aqueous loss as in surgery or trauma.

Doc: describe (deep, moderate, shallow, flat)

- **flare** – protein clumps floating free (circulating, actually) in the aqueous. Associated with inflammation, and often seen after surgery and trauma, and in iritis. Looks like dust falling in the sunlight or hazy like headlights shining through fog.

Doc: note, grade 1+ to 4+ or describe

- **hyphema** (see Figure 5-7B) – blood in the AC/aqueous. Usually settles at the bottom of chamber. Entire chamber may be full and this is called an 8-ball hyphema (because it looks like the black 8-ball used in pool).

Doc: note; describe in percentages, fractions, or measure; draw

- **hypopyon** (Figure 5-24) – pus in AC. White or yellowish white, usually settles at bottom of chamber (as in hyphema).

Doc: note; describe in percentage, or describe in fraction; draw

- **vitreous** – looks like strands of egg white in the AC. Often comes through the pupil (prolapses) in aphakes. Occurs after surgery or trauma.

Doc: note, draw

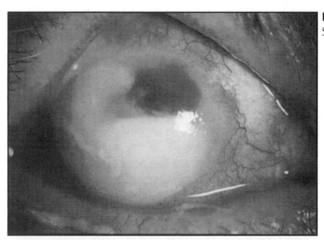

Figure 5-24. Hypopyon. (Photo by Val Sanders.)

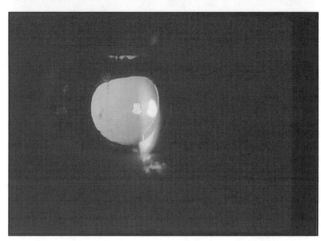

Figure 5-25. Iris atrophy (note area in superior iris where light shines through). (Photo by Val Sanders.)

Iris/Pupil

- **atrophy** (Figure 5-25) – areas of thinned iris, iris may look moth eaten. If you shine the light straight back into the eye and get a red reflex, you can see red shining through the areas of atrophy in the iris. May occur from stretching/tearing during surgery.

Doc: note, give location by the clock, draw

- **coloboma** – congenitally absent wedge of iris, from periphery into pupil. Is usually inferior.

Doc: note, may give location of opening by the clock, draw

- **iris cyst** (Figure 5-26) – a translucent, fluid-filled, raised area or clump on iris surface. (Ultrasound is needed to confirm diagnosis.)

Doc: note, give location, measure, draw

- **iris detachment (iridodialysis)** – root of iris has been torn away from the angle. Viewed well by retroillumination.

Doc: note, describe, give location, draw

- **iris movement (iridodonesis)** – the iris "shakes" when the patient moves the eye. Occurs in aphakes who have no lens to support the iris.

Doc: note

Figure 5-26. Iris cyst (note curve of beam where it hits the cyst). (Photo by Val Sanders.)

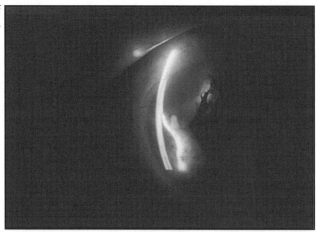

Figure 5-27. Peripheral iridectomy. (Photo by Val Sanders.)

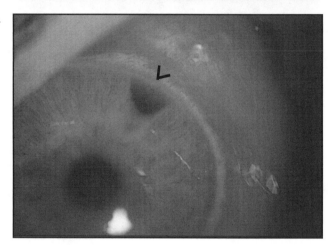

- **iris nevus** – dark freckle (with feathered border) on iris surface; may be flat or slightly raised.

Doc: note, describe, give location, measure, draw

- **iris strands** – this looks like a little wispy hair coming off the iris and waving around in the aqueous. Sometimes the "hair" may have a blob of pigment stuck to it.

Doc: note, draw

- **laser iridotomy** – dot or area of iris that has been opened with laser. Is within iris, not at periphery (as in peripheral iridectomy, below).

Doc: note, give location by the clock, may describe as "patent" or "open" if unoccluded (these sometimes close; light will reflect through if open), draw

- **normal iris vessels** – iris vessels are not usually seen in the heavily pigmented iris. In light eyes they may be visible, but will coincide with the iris pattern and appear to be covered by a membrane. (Just because you see them does not mean it is rubeosis. In a healthy eye, it is probably just a prominent, normal vessel.)

Doc: note, give location by the clock, draw

- **peripheral iridectomy** (Figure 5-27) – wedge cut out of iris during surgery. Usually superior.

Doc: note, give location by the clock, may describe as "patent" or "open" if unoccluded (they are not likely to close, though), draw

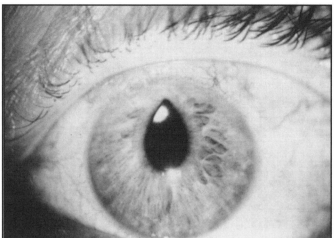

Figure 5-28. Peaked pupil. (Courtesy of Dennis Ryll.)

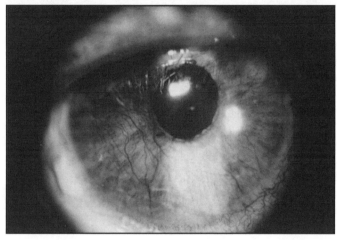

Figure 5-29. Iris rubeosis (note blood vessels on iris). (Courtesy of Dennis Ryll.)

- **pigment dispersion** – area(s) where iris pigmentation is missing.

Doc: note, grade 1+ to 4+

- **pupil reaction** – if the pupil is not dilated, it should react by getting smaller when the light from the slit lamp hits it. If there is no reaction, or the pupil enlarges, this is abnormal.

Doc: note, describe

- **pupil shape** – if the pupil is not round, it is abnormal (Figure 5-28).

Doc: note, describe (ie, "pupil peaked at 2:00"), draw

- **rubeosis** (Figure 5-29) – abnormal blood vessels on the iris surface. Usually seen in diabetes and trauma.

Doc: note, grade 1+ to 4+, draw

- **sector iridectomy** – whole wedge cut out of iris from periphery into pupil. Used to be done during cataract surgery without IOLs. Usually superior.

Doc: note, may give location of opening by the clock, draw

- **synechia** – portion of iris is stuck like glue onto the lens (posterior; Figure 5-30A) or back of cornea (anterior; Figure 5-30B). May see muscle fibers stretching from iris to other structure. If stuck to lens, the pupil margin may be irregular, and the eye may not dilate normally.

Doc: note if anterior or posterior, give location by the clock

Figure 5-30A. Posterior synechia (note adhesions at carets). (Photo by Val Sanders.)

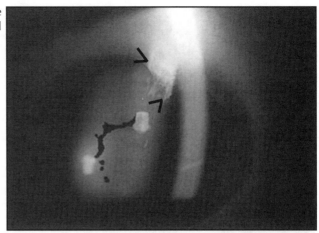

Figure 5-30B. Anterior synechia (note adhesion at caret). (Photo by Val Sanders.)

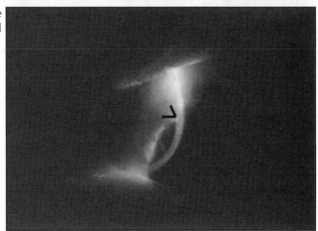

Lens/Intralocular Lens

- **capsule opacity** – white cloud on membrane behind IOL. May be general haze or may be only in a particular spot.

Doc: note, grade density 1+ to 4+, give location by the clock, note whether or not optic zone is clear, draw

- **capsulotomy** (Figure 5-31) – lasered hole in the posterior capsule. If pupil is not dilated and you do not know that the patient has had a capsulotomy, it can be hard to tell if a capsulotomy has been done. Everything behind the IOL looks black (same as a clear capsule). When dilated, it is easy to see the edges of the capsulotomy. Every now and then the capsulotomy hole is not central, and the optic zone still has an opacity.

Doc: note, may describe as "patent" if it is open (although they do not close), comment if optic zone is still obstructed, draw

- **cataract** – general term for any opacification of the lens (Table 5-8).

Doc: note, describe (including shape, texture, and color), give location, tell if optic axis is affected, grade density 1+ to 4+, draw

- **cortical cataract** – whitish lines, dots, or streaks (spokes) in the lens cortex. May be arrow-shaped (wider at the periphery, point at center) or like spokes of a wheel. Spokes may be

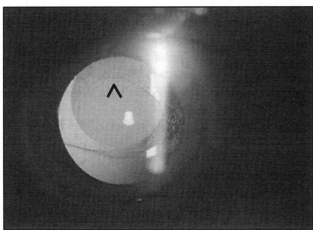

Figure 5-31. Patent posterior capsulotomy (note edge of opening at caret). (Photo by Val Sanders.)

TABLE 5-8
Types of Cataracts*

Type of Cataract	Localization and Appearance	Comments
Congenital (formed in utero or during infancy)		
1. Polar	Anterior or posterior (axial area) of the lens capsule; appears as fine white dots	Usually hereditary; commonly remains stationary throughout life; visual acuity is only affected if opacity is large
2. Zonular (Lamellar)	Gray round opacities surrounded by a dark, clear zone; can occur in pre- or postnatal development	Hereditary; usually occurs bilaterally; has tendency to increase in size during 3rd to 5th decade
Presenile (formed during early childhood/young adulthood)		
1. Coronary	Wreath of opacities in periphery of cortex	Appears in puberty; inherited; need widely dilated pupil to view, vision rarely affected
Senile (appearance generally following ages 30 to 40)		
1. Nuclear Sclerosis (NS)	Lens nucleus normally hardens with age; index of refraction of nucleus increases, inducing myopia; the world appears "yellower" as the lens acts as a filter for blue wavelengths	Myopic changes in Rx ("second sight"); slow, gradual reduction in vision
2. Cortical (Cort)	Cortex absorbs water and swells, creating radial opacities (waterclefts); can progress to form cortical spokes	Can occur in combination with other senile lens changes
3. Posterior Subcapsular (PSC)	Opacity on the posterior capsular face; appears along optical axis or just inferiorly	Appears as dark irregularity in retroillumination; glare, especially at night, is common complaint; this type can be most visually impairing due to its axial placement and density
Toxic or Complicated		
1. Steriods	Typically PSC types	
2. Miotics (PI, DFP)	Anterior subcapsular opacities	
3. Infrared (glass blower's)	Anterior lens capsule exfoliation	
4. Copper (chalasis)	Sunflower cataract in subcapsular cortex	
5. Iron (siderosis)	Brownish subcapsular opacity	
6. X-rays	PSC type	
7. Chronic inflammation	PSC type	

*Adapted with permission from Nemeth SC, Shea CA. *Medical Sciences for the Ophthalmic Assistant*. rev. ed. Thorofare, NJ; SLACK Incorporated; 1991.

TABLE 5-9
Grading Cortical Cataracts

Feature	Grade
Gray lines, dots, and flakes aligned along the cortical fibers in periphery; visible in oblique direct illumination.	1+ (early or incipient)
Opaque spokes, anterior chamber may be shallower than normal for patient	2+ (immature or intumescent)
Cortex opaque up to capsule, anterior chamber may again be normal depth	3+ (mature)
Lens is smaller, wrinkly capsule, nucleus may float in liquefied cortex	4+ (hypermature)

Figure 5-32. Nuclear sclerotic cataract. (Photo by Val Sanders.)

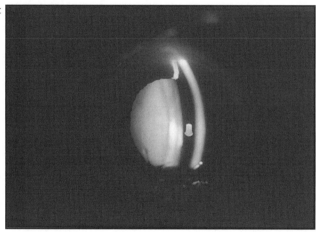

so peripheral that they are only seen when dilated. Eventually cortex may liquefy and nucleus "floats".

Doc: note, grade 1+ to 4+ (Table 5-9), describe location by the clock, note if spoke extends into the optic zone, draw

- **intraocular lens** (IOL) – plastic implant inserted during or after cataract surgery. If the lens is in front of the iris, it is an AC lens. If the lens is AC but clipped into the iris (with pegs or clips), it is an iris plane. An IOL behind the iris and pupil is a PC lens. The lens should be centered, but rarely they slip or drift (this is best seen after dilation).

Doc: note according to location (AC, iris plane, PC), type (if known), centration (note, draw)

- **nuclear sclerosis** (Figure 5-32) – generalized yellowing of the lens. If the color is more brownish, it is termed "brunescent." If totally white and opaque, it is "mature."

Doc: note, grade 1+ to 4+ (Table 5-10), note color abnormalities

- **opacity** – any cloudy area.

Doc: note, describe (color, size, location), draw

- **posterior subcapsular cataract** (Figure 5-33) – whitish opacity on the far back part of the lens. Can be hard to see (especially if you are trying to see through nuclear sclerosis). May be best viewed in retroillumination.

Doc: note, grade 1+ to 4+ (Table 5-11)

TABLE 5-10
Grading Nuclear Sclerotic Cataracts

Lens Color	Grade
Gray-blue (normal)	0
Yellow overtone	1+
Light amber	2+
Reddish brown	3+
Brown or black, opaque, no fundus reflection	4+

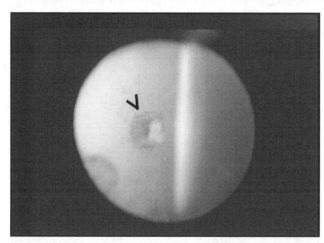

Figure 5-33. Posterior subcapsular cataract. (Photo by Val Sanders.)

TABLE 5-11
Grading Posterior Subcapsular Cataracts

Feature	Grade
Optical irregularity on posterior capsule; visible only on retroillumination	1+
Small, white fleck	2+ (early)
Enlarged plaque; round or irregular borders	3+ (moderate)
Opaque plaque	4+ (advanced)

- **precipitates** (Figure 5-34) – brown dots, or may be a fine brown weblike deposit on IOL.

Doc: note, grade 1+ to 4+

- **pseudoexfoliation** (Figure 5-35) – gray dandrufflike flecks on lens (may also appear on pupillary margin).

Doc: note, grade 1+ to 4+, give location

- **subluxation** – the lens has slipped out of place partially or entirely.

Doc: note, describe, draw

Figure 5-34. Precipitates on an IOL implant. (Photo by Val Sanders.)

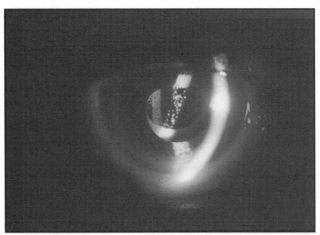

Figure 5-35. Pseudoexfoliation. (Photo by Val Sanders.)

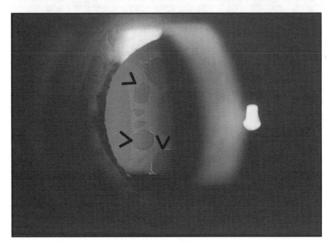

- **vacuoles** – look like little bubbles in the lens.

Doc: note, draw

Vitreous

- **asteroid hyalosis** – small, yellow, oval opacities (called miscelles) "stuck" in the vitreous gel. Highly reflective calcium, usually occurs in one eye only.

Doc: note, grade 1+ to 4+

- **opacities** – often golden, yellow, or white. May be red or white blood cells, cholesterol, or calcium. Best seen through dilated pupil.

Doc: note, describe

- **syneresis scintillans** – small, angular, golden crystals that float freely in the vitreous. Usually occurs in both eyes, often related to vitreous degeneration/liquification (syneresis) or old trauma.

Doc: note, grade 1+ to 4+

- **vitreous strands** – look like strands of eggwhite in the anterior chamber. May be floating through the pupil, still attached to the vitreous face. May run to wound site (internally).

Doc: note, describe, draw

Chapter 6

The Problematic Examination

- Many systemic diseases cause eye problems that can be detected with the slit lamp.

- Even if a systemic condition itself does not directly affect the eye, the eye may be affected by medication taken for that condition.

- There is the possibility of a local allergic reaction with virtually any topical ocular medication.

You glance at the patient's chart before calling her back. This is a follow-up exam for dry eye. What should you be especially looking for on her slit lamp exam? The first section of this chapter lists common ocular diseases and conditions with specifics to be cognizant of as you do the microscopic evaluation. The second section covers common ocular trauma.

The next patient in your exam chair gives a history of gout, for which he is taking allopurinol. Did you know that these can affect what you see during the slit lamp exam? The third part of this chapter lists systemic diseases and conditions in alphabetical order, followed by possible slit lamp findings. In the fourth section, systemic medications are listed by both generic and trade names, with details on potential microscopic affects. Finally, the fifth section lists topical ocular medications (by generic name, trade name, and sometimes category) and their possible slit lamp detectable side effects. For the patient mentioned above, you would look for episcleritis, scleritis, corneal crystals, and iritis associated with the inflammatory process in gout. You would also watch for cataracts, a possible side effect of allopurinol. Take a thorough history, identify possible ocular findings, and offer your patients the most careful slit lamp examination available!

Ocular Diseases and Conditions

Notes:
> *Some of the possible findings are admittedly rare.*
> *Some of the possible findings may be absent in a particular patient or case.*
> *See also notes on medications used to treat these conditions.*

- **blepharitis:** chalazion formation, collarettes, crusting/matting, lid edema, lid erythema, froth, lash loss, lid notching, packed meibomian glands, trichiasis, decreased tear BUT, debris in tear film, matter, oily tear film, conjunctival dryness, conjunctival injection, stained corneal dry spots, punctate epithelial erosions.
- **cellulitis:** lid edema, lid erythema.
- **conjunctivitis:** crusting/matting, debris in tear film, epiphora, matter, oily tear film, conjunctival edema, follicles, conjunctival injection, papillae, punctate epithelial erosions/stained areas.
- **contact dermatitis:** lid edema, lid erythema, lid rash, tissue sloughing.
- **corneal dystrophy:** corneal edema, corneal opacities, increasing corneal thickness, vascularization, bullae, recurrent epithelial erosion.
- **dacryocystitis:** redness medial to inner canthus, swelling medial to inner canthus, crusting/matting, epiphora, matter, reflux.
- **dry eye syndrome:** blepharitis, lid position (lower puncta may not contact globe), decreased tear BUT, debris in tear film, oily tear film, conjunctival dryness, conjunctival injection, stained corneal dry spots, desiccated tissue (stains with rose bengal).
- **ectropion:** lower puncta does not contact globe, epiphora, injection of palpebral conjunctiva, conjunctival dryness (inferior), conjunctival injection, stained corneal dry spots.
- **endophthalmitis:** lid edema and spasms, conjunctival erythema, conjunctival chemosis, corneal edema, marked anterior chamber reaction that may include an hypopyon.
- **entropion:** trichiasis, reduced tear production, conjunctival injection, corneal abrasions/keratitis (from lashes rubbing cornea), corneal scarring, corneal ulcer.
- **episcleritis** (Figure 6-1): increased tearing, episcleral injection (redness of vessels deeper than the conjunctiva, do not bleach on instillation of phenylephrine); red, blue, or purple

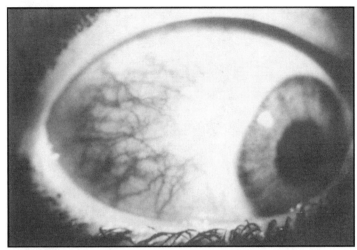

Figure 6-1. Episcleritis (note raised nodule). (Reprinted with permission from *Medical Sciences for the Ophthalmic Assistant,* SLACK Incorporated.)

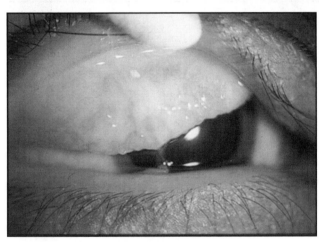

Figure 6-2. Giant papillary conjunctivitis. (Photo by Val Sanders.)

raised nodule; conjunctival/episcleral salmon-pink patch; corneal dellen; corneal edema; infiltrates.

- **exophthalmus:** incomplete lid closure, lid lag, lid malposition, epiphora, conjunctival dryness, scleral show, stained corneal dry spots (see also associated causative disorders).
- **giant papillary conjunctivitis** (Figure 6-2)**:** mucus discharge, papillae on palpebral conjunctiva of upper lid.
- **Herpes simplex:** lid lesions (primary), follicles, watery discharge, conjunctival injection, corneal dendrite, corneal edema, corneal scarring.
- **iritis (anterior uveitis,** Figure 6-3)**:** ciliary flush, keratitic precipitates, cell and flare in anterior chamber, miotic pupil, posterior synechiae.
- **keratitis (inflammatory disorder):** decreased tear BUT, watery or purulent discharge, conjunctival injection, conjunctivitis, corneal dry spots, corneal infiltrates, corneal ulcer, corneal staining.
- **keratoconus (ectatic corneal dystrophy):** lower lid distended by corneal cone in downgaze, blue sclera, central corneal thinning, corneal scarring, vertical striae, Fleischer ring, visible stromal nerves, breaks in endothelium and/or Descemet's membrane, corneal edema.

Figure 6-3. Classic signs of iritis, with ciliary injection, tearing, and miosis. (Reprinted with permission from *Medical Sciences for the Ophthalmic Assistant*, SLACK Incorporated.)

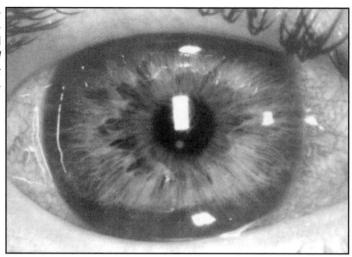

- **keratopathy (noninflammatory disorder):** lid malposition, incomplete lid closure, band keratopathy, bullae, corneal edema, filaments, striae.
- **nasolacrimal obstruction:** crusting/matting, epiphora, matter, reflux.
- **open angle glaucoma:** anterior chamber depth, angle openings.
- **pigmentary glaucoma:** Krukenberg spindles; other pigment on corneal endothelium; slit-like openings in the mid periphery of the iris, visible with retroillumiation.
- **recurrent erosion syndrome:** epiphora, conjunctival injection, corneal edema (localized), irregular corneal surface, corneal staining, corneal scarring, corneal ulcer.
- **scleritis:** conjunctival and episcleral injection, deep violet discoloration in affected area (does not bleach with topical phenylephrine), increased vascularity visible with green filter, scleral thinning, corneal opacities, corneal edema, anterior chamber inflammation (cells and flare).
- **uveitis (posterior):** hypopyon.

Ocular Trauma

Notes:
Some of the findings are rare but are entities that you should watch out for.
Findings will vary from case to case.
Infection is always possible after a penetrating injury or corneal compromise.
For postoperative findings, see Chapter 7.

- **black eye:** bruising, lid edema, lid erythema, epiphora, conjunctival injection, subconjunctival hemorrhage, corneal abrasion, anterior chamber reaction (cell and flare), hyphema, torn iris, lens subluxation, traumatic cataract.
- **chemical burn:** blepharospasm, lid edema, lid erythema, blistered skin, epiphora, conjunctival chemosis, conjunctival injection, conjunctivitis, corneal abrasion, corneal edema, keratitis, corneal staining, iritis.
  Possible later: lid scarring, entropion, trichiasis, recurrent corneal erosion, corneal scarring, dry eye.

- **conjunctival laceration:** blepharospasm, conjunctival chemosis, conjunctival injection, subconjunctival hemorrhage.
- **corneal abrasion:** blepharospasm, foreign body on palpebral conjunctiva, foreign body in fornix, epiphora, conjunctival injection, corneal staining, striae, anterior chamber reaction (cell and flare).
  Possible later: corneal edema, corneal scarring, recurrent erosion syndrome, iritis.
- **foreign body (corneal):** blepharospasm, epiphora, conjunctival injection, conjunctival laceration, corneal abrasion, corneal edema, infiltrates, rust ring (if foreign body was metallic), striae, corneal perforation, anterior chamber reaction (cell and flare).
  Possible later: corneal scar, recurrent corneal erosion, iritis.
- **lid laceration:** blepharospasm, bruising, lid edema, lid erythema.
  Possible later: epiphora, lid scarring, trichiasis, entropion, ectropion.
- **perforated globe:** blepharospasm, epiphora, conjunctival chemosis, conjunctival injection, subconjunctival hemorrhage, uveal prolapse, corneal edema, anterior chamber reaction (cell and flare), hyphema, lens subluxation, traumatic cataract.
- **radiation (ultraviolet) burn:** blepharospasm, lid edema, lid erythema, blistered skin, epiphora, conjunctival injection, keratitis, corneal staining, iritis.
  Possible later: recurrent corneal erosion.
- **thermal burn- of lids:** blepharospasm, lid edema, lid erythema, blistered skin; **of cornea:** blepharospasm, epiphora, conjunctival chemosis, conjunctival injection, corneal abrasion/burn, corneal edema, keratitis, corneal staining, anterior chamber reaction (cell and flare).
  *Possible later: **lids-** lid scarring, trichiasis, entropion; **cornea-** corneal scarring, recurrent corneal erosion, iritis.*

Systemic Diseases and Conditions

Notes:
  Some of these findings are admittedly rare.
  "Conjunctivitis" can include conjunctival redness, conjunctival edema, excessive tearing, and matter/discharge.
  See also notes on medications used to treat these conditions.

- **abuse (physical):** lid bruises and swelling, lid burns, subconjunctival hemorrhage (may be numerous and tiny), corneal abrasion, hyphema, traumatic cataract, lens subluxation.
- **acne:** (see Rosacea).
- **Acquired Immune Deficiency Syndrome (AIDS):** exophthalmus; conjunctivitis (recurrent infections); dry eye; Kaposi's sarcoma (reddish-blue vascular nodules) of lids, palpebral conjunctiva, or conjunctiva.
- **albinism:** nystagmus, white brows and lashes, reddish iris.
- **alcoholism:** ptosis, nystagmus, iris paralysis.
- **allergies:** conjunctivitis, congestion of conjunctival blood vessels, dry eye (secondary to medication), iritis (seasonal).
- **anemia:** subconjunctival hemorrhage.
- **ankylosing spondylitis:** iritis.
- **arteriosclerosis:** arcus senilis.

- **asthma:** conjunctivitis, cataract (secondary to corticosteroid treatment).
- **Bell's Palsy:** incomplete or absent lid closure, exposure keratitis.
- **breast cancer:** metastatic lesion to angle, metastatic lesion to iris, other metastatic lesions (visible mass, redness), symptoms of metastatic lesions (exophthalmus, hyphema).

OphA

- **cancer** (see Breast Cancer, Colon Cancer, Leukemia, Lung Cancer, Melanoma).
- **Candida albicans (yeast):** swelling of lacrimal gland, lid "thrush," conjunctivitis, stringy mucus, keratitis, pseudomembranes.
- **carotid artery disease:** dilation of conjunctival blood vessels, iritis.

OphA

- **chickenpox:** vesicles on lid, conjunctivitis, abnormal pupil, superficial punctate keratitis, iritis.
- **Chlamydia:** lid swelling, conjunctival injection, conjunctivitis, conjunctival pseudomembranes, keratitis, corneal vascularization.
- **colon cancer:** metastatic lesions (visible mass, redness), symptoms of metastatic lesions (exophthalmus, hyphema).
- **craniofacial syndromes:** exophthalmus, nystagmus, exposure keratitis, coloboma.

OphA

- **diabetes:** xanthelasma, corneal wrinkles, rubeosis of iris, loss of iris pigment, cataract, asteroid hyalosis.
- **Downs Syndrome:** nystagmus, epicanthal folds, keratoconus, iris spots, Brushfield's spots (gray or white spots around the edge of the iris), cataract.
- **eczema:** lid crusting, scaling, and oozing (blepharitis); conjunctivitis; conjunctival thickening; congestion of conjunctival blood vessels; dry eye; keratoconus; cataract.
- **emphysema:** cataract (secondary to corticosteroid treatment).
- **endocarditis:** nystagmus, tiny red dots on conjunctiva, anisocoria, iritis.
- **facial deformity syndromes:** microphthalmos, down-sloping lid slant, nystagmus, lower lid coloboma, dermoid cysts of the globe, cataract.
- **German measles (congenital defects following maternal infection):** microphthalmos, nystagmus, corneal edema, corneal clouding, iris atrophy, aniridia, cataract.
- **German measles (acute postnatal cases):** follicular conjunctivitis.

OphA

- **gonorrhea (neonatorum):** edema of orbit, lid edema, congestion of conjunctival blood vessels, conjunctival chemosis, purulent conjunctivitis, conjunctival pseudomembranes, keratitis, corneal perforation, iritis.
- **gout:** episcleritis, scleritis, corneal crystals, iritis.
- **hay fever:** conjunctivitis, congestion of conjunctival blood vessels, dry eye (secondary to medication), iritis (seasonal).
- **Herpes simplex (congenital defects following maternal infection):** cataract.

OphA

- **Herpes simplex (acute postnatal cases):** lid lesions, follicular conjunctivitis, limbal dendrites, corneal dendrites, corneal edema.
- **Herpes zoster** (see Shingles).
- **histoplasmosis:** conjunctivitis.

OphA

- **hypertension:** arcus senilis.
- **hypervitaminosis A, B, and D:** exophthalmus, calcium deposits in conjunctiva (D), band keratopathy (D), cataract (D).

OphA

- **influenza:** keratitis.
- **leprosy:** lash loss (brows and lids), paralysis of lid, thickened corneal nerves, corneal pannus, corneal scarring, corneal perforation, keratitis, iritis, iris nodules, cataract.

- **leukemia:** exophthalmus, metastatic lesions (visible mass, redness), symptoms of metastatic lesions (exophthalmus, hyphema).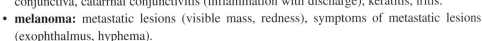
- **lung cancer:** metastatic lesion to angle, metastatic lesion to iris, other metastatic lesions (visible mass, redness), symptoms of metastatic lesions (exophthalmus, hyphema).
- **lupus:** roundish lesions on lids, congestion of conjunctival blood vessels, episcleritis, keratitis, iridocyclitis.
- **malaria:** conjunctivitis, keratitis, iritis.
- **malnutrition:** lid edema, conjunctival chemosis, dry eye, keratopathy.
- **Marfan's Syndrome:** nystagmus, blue sclera, off-center pupil, multiple pupils, pupillary membrane, subluxed lens.
- **measles:** Koplik's spot (tiny white grain surrounded by a red round area) on caruncle or conjunctiva, catarrhal conjunctivitis (inflammation with discharge), keratitis, iritis.
- **melanoma:** metastatic lesions (visible mass, redness), symptoms of metastatic lesions (exophthalmus, hyphema).
- **menopause:** increased wrinkling of skin, ectropion, entropion, ptosis, dermatochalasis, dry eye.
- **mononucleosis:** swelling indicating infection of the lacrimal gland, lid edema, conjunctivitis.
- **multiple sclerosis:** nystagmus, ptosis, anisocoria.
- **mumps:** swelling indicating infection of the lacrimal gland, conjunctivitis, episcleritis, scleritis, unilateral keratitis, stromal keratitis and vascularization (interstitial keratitis), iritis.
- **muscular dystrophy disorders:** ptosis, dry eye, cataract.
- **myasthenia gravis:** ptosis, abnormal pupil.
- **neurofibromatosis (von Recklinghausen's Disease):** exophthalmus, thickened lid margins, lid neurofibroma, cafe au lait marks on lids, ptosis, limbal neurofibroma, prominent corneal nerves, iris nodules.
- **occlusive vascular disorder (progressive):** dilation of conjunctival vessels, iritis.
- **parathyroid (overactive):** calcification of conjunctiva, corneal opacities (calcium deposits), band keratopathy.
- **parathyroid (underactive):** blepharospasm, conjunctivitis, keratitis, cataract.
- **Parkinson's Disease:** eyelid tremors, diminished blinking.
- **peptic ulcer disease:** iritis.
- **psoriasis:** scaling lid skin, blepharitis, exfoliated scales in conjunctival sac, conjunctivitis, corneal infiltrates, corneal erosion, corneal vascularization.
- **rheumatoid arthritis:** conjunctivitis, dry eye, episcleritis, scleritis, scleral thinning, keratitis sicca, band keratopathy, corneal melting, iritis, cataract.
- **rosacea:** blepharitis, conjunctivitis, multiple chalazia, keratitis, corneal ulcers, corneal infiltrates, corneal pannus, iritis.
- **rubeola** (see Measles).
- **rubella** (see German Measles).
- **sarcoidosis:** swelling of lacrimal gland, sarcoid lid nodule, episcleral nodule, keratitic precipitates, corneal edema, iritis.
- **scleroderma:** scarring of lid margin, keratitis, corneal ulceration, cataract.
- **shingles (Herpes zoster):** vesicles on lid, ptosis, lid edema, lid redness, incomplete lid closure, scleritis, keratitis, exposure keratitis, corneal edema, infiltrates, iritis.
- **Sickle Cell Disease:** comma-shaped conjunctival vessels.

- **sinus problems:** conjunctivitis, congestion of conjunctival blood vessels, dry eye (secondary to medication), iritis (seasonal).
- **smallpox:** lid lesions, trichiasis, symblepharon (lid adheres to the globe), conjunctivitis, severe keratitis, leukoma (white corneal opacity), iritis, patchy iris atrophy, vitreous opacity.
- **smoking:** dry eye, cataract.
- **temporal (cranial) arteritis:** iritis.
- **temporal (giant cell) arteritis:** ptosis, iritis.
- **third nerve palsy (oculomotor nerve palsy):** ptosis, anisocoria.
- **thyroid (overactive):** exophthalmus, orbital puffiness, lid retraction, lid lag, incomplete lid closure, exposure keratitis, keratoconjunctivitis of superior limbus.
- **thyroid (underactive):** periorbital edema, loss of outer third of brows, lid edema, mild cortical lens opacities.
- **toxoplasmosis (congenital and acquired):** conjunctivitis, leukokoria ("white pupil"), vitreous haze.
- **tuberculosis:** scleritis, phlyctenular keratoconjunctivitis (tiny red pustules on conjunctiva and/or cornea).
- **vaccinia:** lid infection, cellulitis, lid vesicles, blepharitis, conjunctivitis, keratitis, corneal perforation, vitreous opacity.
- **varicella** (see Chickenpox).
- **variola** (see Smallpox).
- **Vitamin A deficiency:** foamy patches on bulbar conjunctiva, conjunctival dryness, corneal dryness, corneal haze, corneal perforation.
- **Vitamin B deficiency:** conjunctival dryness, corneal dryness.
- **Vitamin C deficiency:** subconjunctival hemorrhage.

Systemic Medications

Notes:
> *Some of these findings are admittedly rare.*
> *"Conjunctivitis" can include conjunctival redness, conjunctival edema, excessive tearing, and matter/discharge.*
> *Drugs are listed by generic and trade names.*
> *An asterisk (*) indicates an incidence of 3% or more for that particular side effect.*
> *Some trademark drugs are listed because they fall into a category of drug that can cause certain findings, and the findings listed may apply to the category as a whole. This list is intended to be used as a guide. Consult a drug reference book for more information.*

- **Abilify™:** conjunctivitis, dry eye, increased tearing.
- **Accutane™:** eyelid inflammation, dry eye, conjunctivitis, contact lens intolerance, corneal opacity, keratitis, cataract, fetal microphthalmia.
- **Acifex™:** dry eye, corneal opacity, cataract.
- **Actonel™:** dry eye*, conjunctivitis*, cataract*
- **Advair™:** dry eye, redness*, conjunctivitis*, ocular infection*, keratitis* cataract
- **Aerobid™:** ocular infection.
- **Aldoril ™:** Bell's Palsy.

- **allopurinol:** cataract.
- **Altoprev™:** Bell's Palsy*, lens opacity/changes.
- **Ambien™:** scleritis, corneal ulceration.
- **amiodarone:** keratopathy, corneal opacity, corneal degeneration, lens opacities.
- **amphetamines:** widened lid fissures, mydriasis.
- **antibiotics (systemic):** conjunctivitis, keratitis.
- **anticoagulants:** subconjunctival hemorrhage.
- **antidepressants:** cycloplegia, mydriasis.
- **antihistamines:** cycloplegia, mydriasis.
- **Aralen™:** whitening of lashes, ptosis, palpebral edema, deposits in cornea (subepithelial), corneal changes, loss of foveal reflex.
- **Arava™:** conjunctivitis*.
- **Aricept™:** blepharitis, dry eye, cataract.
- **Aristocort™ (contains corticosteroids):** exophthalmos, ptosis, mydriasis, posterior sub-capsular cataract.
- **atropine:** decreased tearing, mydriasis.
- **Atrovent™:** conjunctivitis, precipitate angle closure.
- **Avapro™:** conjunctivitis.
- **Azmacort™ (inhaler/nasal spray, contains corticosteroids):** exophthalmos, ptosis, mydriasis, posterior subcapsular cataract.
- **Bactrim™:** exudative conjunctivitis, iritis.
- **Bentyl™:** mydriasis.
- **Bextra™:** dry eye, subconjunctival hemorrhage, cataract.
- **barbiturates:** ptosis, nystagmus, dermatitis (lids), conjunctivitis, mydriasis, miosis.
- **Botox™:** lagophthalmos, ptosis*, lid edema, entropion, corneal ulceration, keratitis, precipitate angle closure.
- **caffeine:** blepharospasm, tearing*.
- **Catapres™:** dry eye.
- **Celebrex™:** conjunctivitis, cataract.
- **Celexa™:** ptosis, abnormal tearing, dry eye, conjunctivitis, keratitis, mydriasis, cataract
- **CellCept™:** abnormal tearing*, conjunctivitis*, cataract*.
- **chloroquine:** whitening of lashes, ptosis, deposits in cornea (subepithelial), corneal edema.
- **Cialis™:** lid swelling, increased tearing.
- **Cipro™:** conjunctival edema.
- **Clinoril™:** conjunctivitis.
- **Clozapine™:** ptosis, redness, mydriasis.
- **Combivent™ :** precipitate angle closure.
- **Cordarone™:** keratopathy, corneal opacity, corneal degeneration, lens opacities.
- **corticosteroids (systemic):** exophthalmos, ptosis, mydriasis, posterior subcapsular cataract.
- **Coumadin™:** subconjunctival hemorrhage, cycloplegia, mydriasis.
- **Cozaar™:** cataract*.
- **Cytovene™:** Bell's Palsy, corneal decomposition.
- **Decadron™:** exophthalmos, posterior subcapsular cataract.
- **DepaKote™:** dry eye*, conjunctivitis*.

- **Depo-Medrol™:** periocular inflammation, ocular inflammation.
- **Depo-Provera™:** Bell's Palsy.
- **Detrol™:** dry eye*.
- **Diabinese™:** conjunctivitis, mydriasis.
- **diazepam:** decreased blinking, nystagmus (overdose), conjunctivitis.
- **digitalis preparations:** conjunctivitis.
- **digoxin:** conjunctivitis.
- **Dilantin™:** nystagmus, ptosis, allergic conjunctivitis.
- **Ditropan™:** dry eye*, cycloplegia, mydriasis.
- **Diupres™:** conjunctival injection, congestion of conjunctival blood vessels, miosis, iritis.
- **DuoNeb™:** precipitate angle closure.
- **Effexor™:** exophthalmos, blepharitis, dry eye, conjunctivitis, conjunctival edema, scleritis, subconjunctival hemorrhage, keratitis, miosis, mydriasis.
- **Eldepryl™:** blepharospasm.
- **Estratest™:** contact lens intolerance.
- **Evoxac™:** scleritis, keratoconjunctivitis, corneal ulceration, hyphema, ocular infection, mydriasis.
- **Excedrin Extra-Strength™** (contains caffeine): blepharospasm.
- **Fareston™:** dry eye*, corneal keratopathy.
- **Fazaclo™:** narrow angle glaucoma.
- **Fioricet™** (contains caffeine): blepharospasm.
- **Fiorinal™** (contains caffeine): blepharospasm.
- **Flexeril™:** Bell's Palsy.
- **Flexin™:** irregular lens opacities.
- **Flonase™:** dry eye, conjunctivitis, cataract.
- **Flovent™:** conjunctivitis*, cataract.
- **Fosamax™:** scleritis.
- **Glucotrol XL™:** conjunctivitis.
- **Hivid™:** dry eye, redness, mucopurulent conjunctivitis, scleral discoloration, unequal pupil size.
- **Hydrocortone™:** exophthalmos, posterior subcapsular cataract.
- **hydroxychloroquine:** deposits in cornea (subepithelial).
- **Hyzaar™:** lid edema, conjunctivitis.
- **Imitrex™:** palpebral edema, corneal opacity, keratitis, mydriasis.
- **Inderal™:** dry eye.
- **Indocin™:** corneal deposits.
- **Klonopin™:** dry eye, glassy-eyed appearance.
- **Lanoxin™:** conjunctivitis.
- **Lescol™:** cataract, lens opacity/changes.
- **Leukeran™:** minor irregularities to corneal epithelium.
- **Levaquin™:** cataract, lens opacity/changes.
- **Levitra™:** tearing, conjunctivitis.
- **levodopa:** lid retraction, mydriasis.
- **Lexapro™:** ptosis, dry eye, conjunctivitis, ocular infection, mydriasis.
- **Lipitor™:** dry eye.
- **Lomotil™:** decreased tearing, mydriasis.

- **Lotensin HCT™:** conjunctivitis.
- **MAO inhibitors:** mydriasis.
- **marijuana:** decreased tearing, dilation of conjunctival vessels.
- **Medrol™ (contains corticosteroids):** exophthalmos, ptosis, mydriasis, posterior subcapsular cataract.
- **Mevacor™:** Bell's Palsy, lens opacity/changes.
- **morphine:** miosis.
- **myleran (busulfan):** corneal thinning, unspecified lens changes.
- **Namenda™:** ptosis, dry eye, abnormal tearing, subconjunctival hemorrhage, corneal opacity.
- **Naprosyn™:** periorbital edema, corneal opacity.
- **naproxen:** periorbital edema, corneal opacity.
- **Nardil™:** mydriasis.
- **Nasacort™ (inhaler/nasal spray, contains corticosteroids):** exophthalmos, ptosis, mydriasis, posterior subcapsular cataract.
- **Nasonex™:** conjunctivitis.
- **Neurontin™:** ptosis, lid twitch, lacrimal gland disorders, dry eye, conjunctivitis, conjunctival injection, corneal changes, iritis, miosis, cataract.
- **niacin (nicotinic acid):** proptosis.
- **Nolvadex™:** corneal opacities.
- **Norgesic™ (contains caffeine):** blepharospasm.
- **Norpace™:** dry eye.
- **Norvasc™:** dry eye.
- **oral contraceptives:** nystagmus, corneal edema, steepening of corneal curvature, contact lens intolerance.
- **Ortho-Cyclin™:** contact lens intolerance.
- **Ovral™:** contact lens intolerance.
- **Pacerone™:** dry eye, keratopathy, corneal deposits*, corneal degeneration, lens opacity/changes.
- **Pamelor™:** cycloplegia, mydriasis.
- **Paxil™:** exophthalmos, ptosis, blepharitis, conjunctival edema, conjunctivitis, keratoconjunctivitis, corneal ulceration, cataract, mydriasis.
- **Pediazole™:** scleral injection.
- **penicillamine:** ptosis.
- **phenobarbital:** ptosis, nystagmus, dermatitis (lids), conjunctivitis, mydriasis, miosis.
- **Plaquenil™:** deposits in cornea (subepithelial), corneal changes, corneal opacity, corneal edema, loss of foveal reflex.
- **Plavix™:** conjunctivitis, subconjunctival hemorrhage.
- **Pravachol™:** Bell's Palsy, lens opacity/changes, cataract.
- **prednisone** (see corticosteroids [systemic]).
- **Premarin™:** contact lens intolerance.
- **Prempro™:** contact lens intolerance.
- **Prevacid™:** dry eye, conjunctivitis.
- **Prilosec™:** dry eye.
- **Proglycem™:** eyes roll upward, increased tearing.
- **Prosed™:** decreased tearing, mydriasis.

- **Protonix™:** cataract.
- **Prozac™:** exophthalmos, scleritis, mydriasis, iritis, cataract.
- **Pulmicort™:** ocular infection, cataract.
- **Rebetol™:** conjunctivitis*.
- **Rifadin™:** tear discoloration, contact lens staining.
- **Rifater™:** tear discoloration, contact lens staining.
- **Risperdal™:** dry eye, abnormal tearing, blepharitis.
- **Salagen™:** lid twitch, tearing*, iris cysts.
- **salicylates:** nystagmus, subconjunctival hemorrhage, conjunctivitis, mydriasis.
- **Septra™:** scleral injection.
- **Serevent™:** keratitis.
- **Sinemet™:** lid retraction, mydriasis.
- **Sinequan™:** cycloplegia, mydriasis.
- **Singulair™:** conjunctivitis.
- **Soma™:** mydriasis.
- **Sonata™:** dry eye, tearing, corneal erosion.
- **Soriatane™:** lid deposits, dry eye*, abnormal tearing, conjunctivitis*, corneal ulceration, posterior subcapsular cataract*.
- **streptomycin:** conjunctivitis.
- **sulfonamides:** exudative (oozing) conjunctivitis, iritis.
- **Symmetrel™:** corneal punctate erosion, corneal opacity, corneal edema, keratitis, mydriasis.
- **Tamiflu™:** conjunctivitis.
- **tamoxifen:** corneal opacities.
- **Tegretaol™:** punctate corneal lens opacity.
- **Thioridazine™:** corneal deposits, irregular lens opacities, lenticular deposits, miosis, mydriasis.
- **Thorazine™:** hyperpigmentation (lids, conjunctiva, cornea), miosis, pigment deposits in corneal stroma, pigment deposits on lens.
- **Tofranil™:** cycloplegia, mydriasis.
- **Topamax™:** dry eye, abnormal tearing, conjunctivitis, mydriasis, iritis
- **Toprol XL™:** dry eye.
- **Transderm Scop™:** mydriasis, precipitate angle closure.
- **tricyclic antidepressants:** cycloplegia, mydriasis.
- **Tridione™:** nystagmus, conjunctivitis.
- **Trileptal™:** dry eye, subconjunctival hemorrhage, conjunctival edema, mydriasis
- **Ultram™:** cataract.
- **Uniretic™:** iritis.
- **Valium™:** decreased blinking, nystagmus (overdose).
- **Vaseretic™:** palpebral edema, dry eye.
- **Vasotec™:** dry eye.
- **Viagra™:** palpebral edema, dry eye, redness, conjunctivitis, mydriasis.
- **Viracept™:** iritis.
- **Vitamin A:** exophthalmos, nystagmus, lash loss (brows and lids), blepharoconjunctivitis, conjunctival deposits.
- **Vitamin D:** calcium deposits in conjunctiva, calcium deposits in cornea, band keratopathy.

- **Vioxx™:** conjunctivitis.
- **Vytorin™:** lens opacity/changes.
- **warfarin:** subconjunctival hemorrhage, cycloplegia, mydriasis.
- **Wellbutrin™:** dry eye, mydriasis.
- **Xanax™:** mydriasis.
- **Xeloda™:** keratoconjunctivitis*.
- **Zithromax™:** conjunctivitis.
- **Zocor™:** Bell's Palsy, lens opacity/changes.
- **Zoloft™:** exophthalmos, ptosis, dry eye, abnormal tearing, conjunctivitis, hyphema, cataract, mydriasis.
- **Zyban™:** dry eye, mydriasis.
- **Zyloprim™:** cataract.
- **Zyprexa™:** blepharitis, dry eye, conjunctivitis, ocular inflammation, keratoconjunctivitis, cataract, lens pigmentation, miosis, mydriasis.
- **Zyrtec™:** ptosis, dry eye, conjunctivitis.

Topical Ocular Medications

Notes:

Some of these findings are admittedly rare.

"Conjunctivitis" can include conjunctival redness, conjunctival edema, excessive tearing, matter/discharge.

Nearly any topical medication can cause a local reaction if the patient is allergic to any of the preparation's components. Look for mild to moderate conjunctival injection, marked conjunctival chemosis, stringy white matter, and conjunctival papillae.

When the patient is using an ointment, be sure to examine the tear film for residual medication.

If the patient is using a suspension, medication may precipitate out and stick to lashes, collect in the cul de sac, or be suspended in the tear film.

- **Acular™:** allergic reaction, superficial keratitis, superficial infections.
- **AKBeta™:** ptosis, blepharoconjunctivitis, keratitis.
- **AKPentolate™:** swelling, redness, rash, tearing, dilated pupil.
- **AKPro™:** redness, follicular blepharoconjunctivitis, angle closure, conjunctival deposits, mydriasis, keratitis, corneal deposits.
- **AKTob™** (see antibiotics, topical).
- **Alamast™:** dry eye.
- **Albalon™:** increased tearing, redness, mydriasis, punctate keratitis.
- **Alomide™:** blepharitis, chemosis, dry eye, tearing, discharge, congested blood vessels, crystalline deposits, corneal erosion, corneal ulcer, corneal abrasion, keratopathy, keratitis, cells in the anterior chamber.

- **Alphagan-P™:** lid redness, lid swelling, blepharitis, dry eye, tearing, discharge, redness, conjunctival swelling, conjunctival hemorrhage, allergic reaction, corneal staining/erosion.
- **Alrex™:** lid redness, tearing, discharge, dry eye, redness, secondary ocular infection, keratoconjunctivitis, posterior subcapsular cataract formation, perforation of the globe.
- **antibiotic** (topical): rash, lid edema, redness, conjunctival edema, failure to heal, secondary infection.
- **apraclonidine:** allergic response, elevation of upper lid, lid swelling, crusting of lid, blepharitis, tearing, discharge, conjunctival whitening, conjunctival petechia, congested blood vessels, dry eye, conjunctivitis, conjunctival follicles, conjunctival edema, dryness, mydriasis, keratitis, corneal staining, corneal erosion, corneal infiltrate.
- **Azelastine:** conjunctivitis.
- **Azopt™:** blepharitis, crusting lids, dry eye, discharge, tearing, conjunctivitis, keratoconjunctivitis.
- **Betagan™:** ptosis, blepharoconjunctivitis, keratitis.
- **Betimol™:** blepharitis, ptosis, lid erythema, conjunctival injection, dry eye, corneal staining, keratitis, cataract.
- **Betoptic™:** crusty lashes, inflammation, discharge, tearing, erythema, edema, dry eye, corneal punctate staining, keratitis, anisocoria.
- **betaxolol:** crusty lashes, tearing, discharge, inflammation, redness, edema, dry eye, corneal punctate staining, keratitis, anisocoria.
- **bimatoprost:** increase in skin pigmentation, lid redness, increased eyelash growth, eyelash darkening, blepharitis, discharge, tearing, dry eye, redness, conjunctival swelling, SPK, increase in iris pigmentation, iritis, cataract.
- **Bleph-10™** (see sulfacetamide).
- **Blephamide™** (see sulfacetamide; contains prednisolone, see corticosteroid, topical).
- **brimonidine:** lid redness, lid swelling, blepharitis, dry eye, tearing, discharge, redness, conjunctival swelling, conjunctival hemorrhage, allergic reaction, corneal staining/erosion.
- **brinzolamide:** blepharitis, crusting lids, dry eye, discharge, tearing, conjunctivitis, keratoconjunctivitis.
- **carbachol:** increased tearing, conjunctival injection, miosis.
- **Carbastat™:** increased tearing, conjunctival injection, miosis.
- **carbonic anhydrase inhibitor** (topical): allergic reaction, rash, tearing, dryness, superficial punctate keratopathy.
- **carteolol:** ptosis, tearing, redness, blepharoconjunctivitis, conjunctival swelling, corneal staining.
- **Ciloxan™:** crusting lids, lid edema, congestion of conjunctival blood vessels, precipitates in corneal ulcer being treated, keratopathy, keratitis, tearing, corneal infiltrates.
- **ciprofloxacin:** lid edema, crusting lids, tearing, congestion of conjunctival blood vessels, precipitates in corneal ulcer being treated, keratopathy, keratitis, corneal infiltrates.
- **corticosteroid** (topical): ptosis, delayed wound healing, secondary infection, mydriasis, corneal thinning, iritis, posterior subcapsular cataract. Includes: dexamethasone, fluorometholone, medrysone, prednisolone, hydrocortisone, and rimexolone.
- **Cortisporin™** (contains hydrocortisone, see corticosteroid, topical; see antibiotic, topical).
- **Cosopt™:** lid crusting, lid redness, lid swelling, lid scaling, blepharitis, redness, tearing, dry eye, discharge, conjunctivitis, redness, superficial punctate keratopathy, corneal erosion, lens opacity.

- **Crolom™:** periocular dryness, periocular puffiness, hordeola, tearing, conjunctival injection.
- **cromolyn:** periocular dryness, periocular puffiness, hordeola, tearing, conjunctival injection.
- **Cyclogyl™:** swelling, redness, rash, tearing, dilated pupil.
- **cyclopentolate:** swelling, redness, rash, tearing, dilated pupil.
- **Cyclosporin A:** redness, discharge, tearing.
- **Dendrid™:** lid and ocular edema, corneal clouding, punctate defects of epithelium.
- **dexamethasone** (see corticosteroid, topical).
- **diclofenac:** slowed or delayed healing, keratitis, iritis, hyphema, or other bleeding if used postoperatively, redness if used with soft contact lenses in place.
- **dipivefrin:** redness, follicular blepharoconjunctivitis, angle closure, conjunctival deposits, mydriasis, keratitis, corneal deposits.
- **dorzolamide:** lid crusting, lid redness, lid swelling, lid scaling, blepharitis, redness, tearing, dry eye, discharge, conjunctivitis, redness, superficial punctate keratopathy, corneal erosion, lens opacity.
- **echothiophate:** blepharospasm, conjunctival thickening, tearing, redness, iritis, iris cysts, miosis, lens opacities.
- **Elestat™:** discharge, redness.
- **Epifrin™:** allergic lid reaction, congestion of conjunctival blood vessels, conjunctival deposits.
- **epinephrine:** allergic lid reaction, angle closure, congestion of conjunctival blood vessels, conjunctival deposits or pigmentation, cicatricial pemphigoid (conjunctival blisters that scar), mild dilation, soft contact lenses stained black.
- **Flarex™** (see corticosteroid, topical).
- **fluorometholone:** ptosis, conjunctivitis, redness, secondary bacterial infection, keratitis, corneal ulcers, mydriasis, iritis, posterior subcapsular cataract, perforation of the globe.
- **Fluor-Op™** (contains fluorometholone; see corticosteroid, topical).
- **fluoroquinolone:** lid swelling, tearing, dry eye, discharge, redness, conjunctivitis, conjunctival hemorrhage, keratitis.
- **flurbiprofen:** increased tendency to bleed if used following surgery, subconjunctival hemorrhage, hyphema, iritis.
- **FML™** (contains fluorometholone, see corticosteroid, topical).
- **FML Forte™** (contains fluorometholone; see corticosteroid, topical).
- **FML-S™:** ptosis, conjunctivitis, redness, secondary bacterial infection, keratitis, corneal ulcers, mydriasis, iritis, posterior subcapsular cataract, perforation of the globe.
- **Gatifloxacin:** lid swelling, tearing, dry eye, discharge, redness, conjunctivitis, conjunctival hemorrhage, keratitis.
- **Genoptic™:** conjunctivitis, conjunctival epithelial defects, congestion of conjunctival blood vessels, secondary bacterial or fungal ulcer.
- **Gentacidin™** (see gentamicin).
- **gentamicin** (see also antibiotics, topical)**:** conjunctivitis, conjunctival epithelial defects, congestion of conjunctival blood vessels, secondary bacterial or fungal ulcer.
- **Gentak™** (see antibiotics, topical).
- **Herplex™:** lid and ocular edema, corneal clouding, punctate defects of epithelium.
- **HMS™** (contains medrysone; see corticosteroid, topical).
- **hydrocortisone** (see corticosteroid, topical).

- **idoxuridine:** lid and ocular edema, corneal clouding, punctate defects of epithelium.
- **Inflamase™ Mild or Forte** (contains prednisolone; see corticosteroid, topical).
- **Iopidine™:** allergic response, elevation of upper lid, crusting of lid, blepharitis, lid swelling, discharge, tearing, conjunctival whitening, dryness, dry eye, conjunctival petechia, congested blood vessels, conjunctivitis, conjunctival follicles, conjunctival edema, mydriasis, keratitis, corneal staining, corneal erosion, corneal infiltrate.
- **Isopto Cetamid™:** conjunctivitis, congestion of conjunctival blood vessels, secondary infections.
- **ketorolac tromethamine:** allergic reaction, superficial ocular infections, superficial keratitis.
- **Lacrisert™:** lid edema, stickiness or matting of lashes, redness, corneal abrasion from improper insertion technique.
- **latanoprost:** lid swelling, lid redness, lid crusting, tearing, dry eye, punctate epithelial keratitis, iris pigmentation.
- **levobunolol:** ptosis, blepharoconjunctivitis, keratitis.
- **levocabastine:** rash, lid edema, dry eye, redness, tearing, discharge.
- **levofloxacin:** lid swelling, dry eye
- **Livostin™:** rash, lid edema, dry eye, redness, tearing, discharge
- **lodoxamide:** blepharitis, tearing, discharge, chemosis, congested blood vessels, dry eye, crystalline deposits, corneal erosion, corneal ulcer, corneal abrasion, keratopathy, keratitis, cells in anterior chamber.
- **Lotemax™:** lid redness, tearing, discharge, dry eye, redness, secondary ocular infection, keratoconjunctivitis, posterior subcapsular cataract formation, perforation of the globe.
- **loteprednol:** lid redness, tearing, discharge, dry eye, redness, secondary ocular infection, keratoconjunctivitis, posterior subcapsular cataract formation, perforation of the globe.
- **Lumigan™:** increase in skin pigmentation, lid redness, increased eyelash growth, eyelash darkening, blepharitis, discharge, tearing, dry eye, redness, conjunctival swelling, superficial punctate keratopathy, increase in iris pigmentation, iritis, cataract.
- **Macugen™ injection:** discharge, conjunctival hemorrhage, corneal edema, keratitis, endophthalmitis, anterior chamber inflammation, cataract.
- **Maxitrol™** (see antibiotics, topical; contains dexamethasone, see corticosteroid, topical)
- **medrysone** (see corticosteroid, topical).
- **metipranolol:** dermatitis, blepharitis, tearing, conjunctivitis.
- **moxifloxacin:** tearing, discharge, dry eye, redness, conjunctivitis, subconjunctival hemorrhage, keratitis.
- **Muro 128™:** redness, swelling.
- **naphazoline:** redness (overuse).
- **Naphcon-A™:** redness (overuse), dilated pupil.
- **Natacyn™:** conjunctival chemosis, redness.
- **natamycin:** conjunctival chemosis, redness.
- **neomycin:** allergic reactions, follicular conjunctivitis, keratitis (see also antibiotic, topical)
- **Neosporin™** (see antibiotic, topical).
- **Neo-Synephrine™:** angle closure, subconjunctival hemorrhage, mydriasis.
- **Ocufen™:** increased tendency to bleed if used following surgery, subconjunctival hemorrhage, hyphema, iritis.
- **Ocuflox™:** redness, tearing, dryness.

- **Ocupress™:** ptosis, tearing, congestion of conjunctival blood vessels, conjunctival edema, corneal staining, keratitis.
- **ofloxacin:** redness, tearing, dryness.
- **olopatadine:** lid edema, dry eye, keratitis.
- **Opticrom™:** periocular dryness, periocular puffiness, hordeola, tearing, conjunctival injection.
- **OptiPranolol™:** dermatitis, blepharitis, tearing, conjunctivitis.
- **Optivar™:** conjunctivitis.
- **Patanol™:** lid edema, dry eye, keratitis.
- **pheniramine:** redness (overuse), dilated pupil.
- **phenylephrine:** angle closure, subconjunctival hemorrhage, mydriasis.
- **Phospholine Iodide™:** blepharospasm, tearing, conjunctival thickening, redness, miosis, iritis, iris cysts, lens opacities.
- **pilocarpine:** redness, miosis, lens opacity.
- **Pilopine™ gel** (see also pilocarpine): corneal haze.
- **Poly-Pred™** (see antibiotic, topical; contains prednisolone, see corticosteroid, topical).
- **Polysporin™** (see antibiotic, topical).
- **Polytrim™** (see antibiotic, topical).
- **Pred Forte™** (contains prednisolone, see corticosteroid, topical).
- **Pred-G™** (contains prednisolone, see corticosteroid, topical; see also gentamicin).
- **Pred Mild™** (contains prednisolone; see corticosteroid, topical).
- **prednisolone** (see corticosteroid, topical).
- **preservatives:** allergic reactions, corneal opacity, keratitis.
- **Propine™:** angle closure, redness, conjunctival deposits, follicular conjunctivitis, mydriasis, keratitis, corneal deposits.
- **Quixin™:** lid swelling, dry eye.
- **Rescula™:** lengthening/decreased length of lashes, increased number of lashes, ptosis, blepharitis, pigmentation of eyelids, redness, dry eye, discharge, conjunctivitis, keratitis, corneal edema, corneal opacity, iritis, cataract.
- **Restasis™:** redness, discharge, tearing.
- **rimexolone** (see corticosteroid, topical).
- **sodium chloride:** redness, swelling.
- **sulfacetamide** (topical; a sulfonamide)**:** conjunctivitis, congestion of conjunctival blood vessels, secondary infections.
- **sulfonamide** (topical)**:** allergic reaction, secondary infections.
- **tetrahydrozoline:** redness (overuse), dilated pupil.
- **timolol:** ptosis, lid erythema, blepharitis, conjunctival injection, dry eye, corneal staining, keratitis, cataract.
- **Timoptic™** (see timolol).
- **TobraDex™** (see antibiotic, topical; contains dexamethasone, see corticosteroid, topical).
- **Tobrex™** (see antibiotic, topical).
- **tobramycin:** lid swelling, conjunctival erythema (see also antibiotic, topical).
- **Travatan™:** blepharitis, discharge, tearing, dry eye, redness, subconjunctival hemorrhage, conjunctivitis, keratitis, iris discoloration, cell or flare, cataract.
- **travoprost:** blepharitis, discharge, tearing, dry eye, redness, subconjunctival hemorrhage, conjunctivitis, keratitis, iris discoloration, cell or flare, cataract.

- **trifluridine:** palpebral edema, congested blood vessels, dry eye, superficial punctate keratopathy, epithelial keratopathy, stromal edema.
- **trimethoprim** (see antibiotic, topical).
- **Trusopt™:** rash, tearing, dryness, superficial punctate keratopathy
- **Vasocidin™** (see sulfacetamide; contains prednisolone, see corticosteroid, topical).
- **Vasocon™:** redness (overuse).
- **Vasocon-A™:** redness (overuse).
- **Vexol™:** (see corticosteroid, topical).
- **Vigamox™:** tearing, discharge, dry eye, redness, conjunctivitis, subconjunctival hemorrhage, keratitis.
- **Viroptic™:** palpebral edema, congested blood vessels, dry eye, superficial punctate keratopathy, epithelial keratopathy, stromal edema.
- **Visine™ (original):** redness (overuse), dilated pupil.
- **Visudyne™:** cataract.
- **Vitrasert™:** vitreous implant: keratopathy, corneal dellen, shallow chamber, angle closure, hyphema, cell & flare, synechia, cataract/lens opacities, pellet extrusion, endophthalmitis.
- **Voltaren™:** keratitis, iritis, slowed or delayed healing, hyphema or other bleeding if used postoperatively.
- **Xalatan™:** Lid swelling, lid redness, lid crusting, tearing, dry eye, punctate epithelial keratitis, iris pigmentation
- **Zaditor™:** rash, discharge, dry eye, conjunctivitis, keratitis, mydriasis.
- **Zymar™:** lid swelling, tearing, dry eye, discharge, redness, conjunctivitis, conjunctival hemorrhage, keratitis.

Chapter 7

The Postoperative Eye

- The detection of infection is one of the main elements of the postoperative slit lamp exam.

- Slit lamp findings of infection in any structure or tissue include injection, edema, and purulent discharge.

- The slit lamp is also key in identifying allergic and inflammatory reactions.

Findings in Infection

The slit lamp examination following any type of ocular surgery is mainly performed to detect the presence of infection as early as possible. Signs of infection (in any structure or tissue) are redness (injection), swelling (edema), and purulent discharge. The patient may complain of tenderness and pain. External tissue may be warm to the touch.

Endophthalmitis is the most serious complication of infection following any penetrating surgery or injury. This condition is an infection of the internal ocular tissues and can destroy the eye in a short period of time. Worse yet, endophthalmitis can trigger sympathetic ophthalmia, a situation in which the other eye may also be lost. Slit lamp signs of endophthalmitis include postoperative inflammation that is exaggerated beyond what would normally be expected. In addition, watch for lid edema and spasms, redness, conjunctival chemosis, corneal edema, and a marked anterior chamber reaction that may include an hypopyon. The patient may complain of intense discomfort and light sensitivity. (See Chapter 5 for descriptions of separate findings.)

Reactions to Medication

In addition to monitoring for signs of impending infection, the slit lamp is invaluable in picking up evidence of contact allergies. Such reactions can occur not only from medications but also from other contactants, such as suture material and tape. Signs of an allergic reaction include redness, rash, swelling, tissue sloughing (manifested as keratitis in the cornea), and tearing. The patient may complain of itching or discomfort when drops are instilled.

The components of any medication may cause side effects besides allergic reactions. Consult Chapter 6 for slit lamp findings pertinent to the medicine that your patient is taking.

Oculoplastics

Lid Surgery

Following any type of lid surgery, it is common for the involved area to be swollen (1+ to 2+). Bruising may be extensive and should be rated and noted in the patient's chart. Redness, if present, should be slight. Evaluate the wound for healing, discharge, gap, and broken sutures. Fluorescein should be instilled to evaluate the cornea for any abrasions that may have occurred during or after the procedure. Dry spots or keratitis on the lower third of the cornea may indicate incomplete lid closure.

As the wound heals, continue to evaluate for broken sutures. Be on the alert for irregular or excessive scarring. Lid surgery that involves the lid margin may affect lash growth, so watch for trichiasis. In addition, continue to evaluate for corneal staining. Lid position should be noted as well, especially after surgery involving the levator muscle. Watch for entropion, ectropion, incomplete closure, etc. If the surgery was to remove a growth, monitor for recurrence.

Lacrimal Procedures

The three lacrimal procedures we will be concerned with here are probing, intubation, and dacryocystorhinostomy (DCR). Following any of these procedures, there may be some mild eyelid swelling and redness as well as slight discharge. Check the cornea for abrasions that may have occurred during the procedure. Grade any tearing that is present. If intubation was done, the clear tube may be seen running from the upper to the lower punctum. The tube should run directly from one punctum to the other without a loop. There should not be an anterior chamber reaction. If a DCR involved an external incision, check the site for swelling and broken sutures.

Enucleation

After an eye has been enucleated, 1+ to 2+ lid swelling is normal. If the patient is unable to open the lids, gently lift the upper lid. A clear plastic conformer should be overlying the socket. The conjunctiva will be edematous (2+) and may be very injected (it may look like a piece of raw meat). Sutures will be visible. There should not be any conjunctiva or other material prolapsing between these stitches. A mild mucus (nonpurulent) discharge is normal.

As the eye heals, lid and conjunctival edema dissipates. The socket takes on a more pinkish-red color that matches the color of the bulbar conjunctiva. A very slight discharge may persist due to the glands in the remaining conjunctiva; the tissue should be moist. The conformer is discontinued when the socket is healed; at this point the patient is fit with a prostheses.

Extraocular Muscles

The main slit lamp findings after extraocular muscle surgery are subconjunctival hemorrhage and conjunctival injection. There may be exposed sutures in the conjunctiva, which may account for some of the redness. Make a note of any conjunctival wound gape. A very mild mucus discharge is normal. The appearance of choroidal pigment is abnormal and indicates a scleral perforation. Over time, watch for the development of a dellen. Check the cornea for any abrasion that may have occurred during the procedure.

Cornea

Corneal Transplant

During the early postoperative period following a corneal transplant, a careful slit lamp exam is essential (Figure 7-1). The patient's epithelium will initially look irregular and may frequently be missing. The cornea will look swollen and probably have folds (generally 2+ to 3+) in the stroma. The junction of the donor and recipient bed will appear hazy and lumpy (there is often 1+ to 2+ swelling at the junction site). The anterior chamber may be somewhat shallow but should not be flat. It may be difficult to visualize the anterior chamber through the fresh graft, but an evaluation of cell and flare should be performed on each visit. Initially, it is common to see 2+ to 3+ cells and flare. The sutures should be evaluated to ensure that none are broken. Broken sutures should be identified by referring to the cornea as a clock dial.

Figure 7-1. One day following penetrating keratoplasty. (Photo by Val Sanders.)

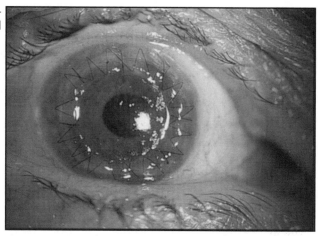

Many physicians will not want topical fluorescein instilled until they have examined the patient. If the epithelium has not healed, the dye may absorb into the stroma, making it impossible to evaluate the extent of corneal healing and anterior chamber reaction. Fluorescein needs to be instilled, however, to check for leaking in the early postoperative course. To evaluate leakage, place a drop of fluorescein into the eye. Instruct the patient to blink once, and then keep the eye open while you observe through the slit lamp. If there is fluid (aqueous) exiting the eye, you will see a tiny clear stream where the fluid is flushing away the stain. Have the patient blink and hold again. If there is a real leak, the stream will reappear. Such leaking indicates wound gap; this is noted as a positive Seidel sign. If there is no leakage, this is recorded as a negative Seidel sign.

As the eye heals, the cornea will gradually take on a normal appearance. Folds will diminish, as will edematous haze. The scar will turn gray, and the graft itself, inside the junction between graft and host, should become clear and thin. The anterior chamber should be more easily visualized.

In addition to infection, the corneal transplant patient must be monitored for rejection. Rejection can occur right after surgery or months (or even years) later. The chief things to look for are corneal edema or haze and the appearance of inflammation in the anterior chamber. Thus, once the eye begins to heal, any increase in cells or flare should be considered as early signs of rejection. The endothelium should be examined for any signs of keratitic precipitates or a linear border (rejection line) of whitish or pigmented opacities running through the graft. The epithelium may become ragged, indicating an epithelial rejection. Epithelial toxicity to topical medication often occurs and presents as punctate keratopathy. Also, any increase in tearing, injection, or ciliary flush at this point can indicate rejection. In addition, you should watch for vascularization forming along sutures. Such neovascularization increases the chances for rejection. (Generally, the patient will verbalize subjective complaints including foreign body sensation, light sensitivity, or discomfort with a rejection episode; therefore, a careful history should be elicited on every exam.)

Pterygium

Injection following the removal of a pterygium may be quite marked. A subconjunctival hemorrhage may also be present. Suture ends may be visible in the conjunctiva. Use fluorescein dye to evaluate for corneal staining (dry spots and superficial punctate keratopathy are common). There may be some corneal edema and striae (1+ to 2+) during the early postoperative period. A

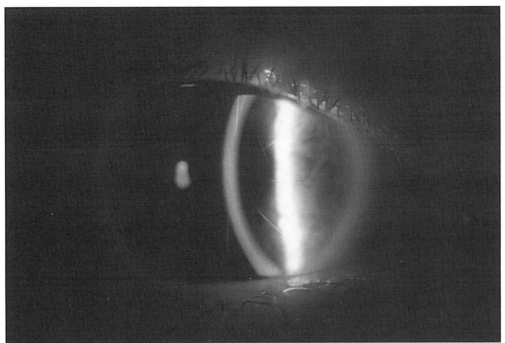

Figure 7-2. Postoperative radial keratotomy. (Photo by Val Sanders.)

mild anterior chamber reaction (1+) may also occur. If a conjunctival graft is used, the borders of the graft should meet the borders of the defect.

Redness may persist for several weeks. Watch for the formation of a dellen (shallow, scooped-out excavation near the limbus) or scleral thinning. Note any corneal scarring. The presence of new vessels at the limbal excision site may indicate the early stages of recurrence.

Refractive Surgery

Incisional refractive surgery is rarely performed for the correction of myopia at this time. The clinician will, however, encounter patients who underwent this procedure in the past. Upon slit lamp examination, one should notice milky thin radial incisions in the anterior to mid stroma (Figure 7-2). Once healed, they should not stain. Today, some surgeons still correct astigmatism with a form of AK (astigmatic keratectomy, Figure 7-3), using either limbal or corneal relaxing incisions. The most common reason for this surgery is to reduce astigmatism at the time of cataract surgery. It may also be performed when laser vision correction is planned and when the patient's astigmatism is greater than the amount approved by the FDA for laser correction. AK incisions are superficial incisions placed parallel to the limbus at the steepest axis of plus cylinder. When first performed, the incisions appear as thin lines of stain. They must be watched for infiltrates, but it is not abnormal to notice a granular appearance in the stroma around the incisions. These are white blood cells in the tissue but are insignificant if they are not organized into clumps or infiltrates.

Excimer laser surgery is performed in two different manners. One is LASIK, which involves a cut corneal flap. The other includes surface treatments (PRK or LASEK), where there is either no flap or the epithelial cells are pushed aside and repositioned after the laser tissue ablation.

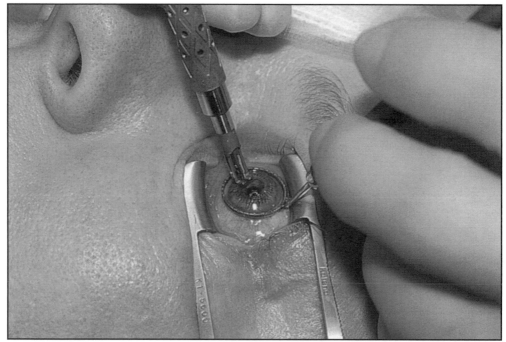

Figure 7-3. Astigmatic keratotomy surgery. (Photo by Val Sanders.)

When examining the patient who has undergone LASIK, one must carefully examine the flap. The flap looks like a circular slice of tissue with an edge left intact. Ideally, it should be difficult to visualize except at the juncture of the flap and the intact peripheral epithelium. The cut edges should be smooth and adhere to the rest of the corneal tissue. Immediate postoperative flap complications are wrinkles, debris under the flap, buttonhole (central thinning or hole), or shifted flap. A centrally grayish jagged area with a clearer center is indicative of a buttonhole or epithelial defect. Occasionally, a flap will become edematous. It will appear milky, and the edges will look lifted. In extreme cases, suturing may be necessary.

When performing the slit lamp exam post LASIK, any irregularity in the epithelium should be noted. As the flap edges heal, one should watch for signs of infection or inflammation. A central haze is not uncommon after any type of excimer treatment, but one should examine the cornea carefully for signs of keratitis. There are two types of keratitis, infectious and toxic. Infectious keratitis can present as anything from mild corneal infiltrates to lamellar abscess formation in the interface. Diffuse lamellar keratitis (DLK) is a noninfectious inflammation that appears like "sand" at the flap interface. It is typically diffuse without extension into the stroma. As it worsens, the clumps of cells begin to look like waves or shifting sand dunes. Severe cases may result in flap melt.

Epithelial ingrowth is a complication usually noted within the first few weeks after a LASIK enhancement, although it may occur after a first treatment as well (Figure 7-4). The appearance varies. It may appear as a clump of graying cells at the flap edge or a swirly pattern into the flap. Occasionally, small cysts or pearls develop. Almost all eyes become dry after LASIK, so they must be monitored for dry spots and punctate keratitis during the slit lamp exam.

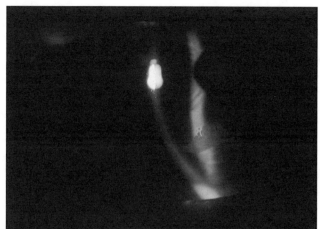

Figure 7-4. Epithelial ingrowth following LASIK. (Photo by Val Sanders.)

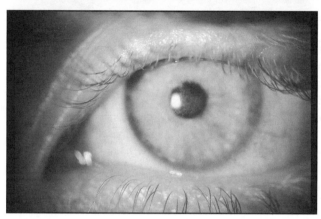

Figure 7-5. Mild anterior stromal haze following LASEK. (Photo by Val Sanders.)

The slit lamp appearance of an eye having undergone a surface treatment is much different than what appears after LASIK. The epithelium is essentially gone after PRK and LASEK. The eye is protected with a bandage contact lens until re-epithelialization occurs. This generally takes 4 to 6 days. During this time, the epithelium is rough and irregular in appearance. One must watch for the appearance of corneal infiltrates and signs of infection during the first few days after surgery. Once the bandage lens is removed, the epithelium must be closely monitored for defects. A faint central stromal haze is usually present to some degree during the first few months after surgery (Figure 7-5) but generally clears by 6 months postoperatively.

Glaucoma

Surgical Trabeculectomy

The slit lamp exam and tonometry are the two tests of concern following a surgical trabeculectomy. Conjunctival injection may be mild to marked (1+ to 3+). There may be a subconjunctival hemorrhage. The conjunctival drainage bleb will usually be large and at least slightly elevated. The suture line is usually superior under the upper cul de sac, so it may be difficult to

Figure 7-6. Filtration bleb. (Photo by Val Sanders.)

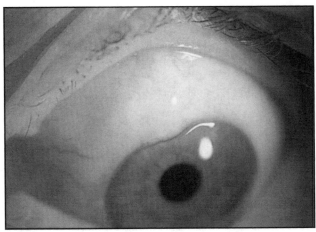

visualize (have the patient look way down). There may be mild corneal edema and/or folds (1+). There is generally a marked anterior chamber reaction of 2+ to 3+. You should also note the chamber depth. Immediately after surgery, it is normal for the chamber to be shallow. Note if a hyphema is present as well as the pupil size and shape. If the trabeculectomy was combined with cataract surgery, see also the section on cataracts.

As the eye heals, continue to monitor the bleb. It should be elevated and blisterlike (Figure 7-6). If not, be sure to note that it is flat. Sometimes a bleb becomes lumpy, cystic, or encapsulated in appearance. Be sure to note if the bleb begins to encroach onto the cornea. Be on the alert for dellen. Watch the AC for depth and inflammation as well as for formation of anterior or posterior synechia. Check the lens for formation of a cataract.

Laser Trabeculoplasty

There may be very mild (1+) conjunctival injection following a laser trabeculoplasty. You may also note the presence of some episcleral congestion. The cornea may evidence some superficial punctate erosions secondary to the contact lens used to direct the laser beam. Transient corneal epithelial burns may also be present. Otherwise, the cornea is generally quiet. Check for anterior chamber reaction, which is usually mild (1+ to 2+). In rare cases, a hyphema may be present. Note the pupil shape and size, and watch for formation of peripheral anterior synechiae.

Laser Iridotomy

Notes on the conjunctiva, cornea, and anterior chamber (including hyphema) given above for laser trabeculoplasty also apply to laser iridotomy. It is important to visualize the iridotomy site itself and to evaluate its patency (ie, that it is open). Iris transillumination is useful for this. If no "glow" is seen through the iridotomy, it is not patent. Indicate the location of the opening with a drawing or by describing it by the clock. Watch for the formation of peripheral anterior synechiae. Evaluate the lens for the presence of isolated opacities (these are permanent).

Cataract

There is more than one way to remove a cataract. However, at the time of this writing, the use of phacoemulsification is most common. In this case, sutures are usually not used. In any event, the following is a general guideline to slit lamp examination following cataract surgery.

Externally, it is normal for some mild lid swelling and ptosis to be evident. Very mild conjunctival injection and chemosis may also be present. You may occasionally see a subconjunctival hemorrhage. Check the wound and note its location. (Most surgeons perform the procedure from the temporal aspect with a 3.00 mm self-sealing incision just anterior to the limbus.) Examine the wound for gape and leak, and check for broken sutures (if the wound was sutured shut). The corneal epithelium may evidence some dry spots or very mild keratitis or staining. (Note: Some physicians may not want fluorescein instilled before they see the patient.) There may be 1+ stromal edema. Folds in Descemet's membrane are not uncommon, perhaps up to 2+. Sometimes, a localized detachment of the endothelium occurs; the membrane balloons away from the cornea and toward the iris. Most of these findings should disappear during the first 1 to 2 weeks after surgery.

There is generally some anterior chamber reaction, often from 1+ to 2+. Check chamber depth. The chamber should be well formed and not flat. Some patients tend to bleed more than others, and you might see an occasional hyphema. There should not be any vitreous in the AC, but if there is, it looks like strands of egg white. Make a note regarding the pupil's size and shape.

Check to see that the IOL is in place, if one was implanted. If the IOL is placed properly, the slit lamp reflex visible on the IOL should be parallel to the plane of the iris. You should not be able to see the haptics or the edge of a posterior chamber IOL (unless the pupil is dilated). Examine the IOL surface for the presence of precipitates during the postoperative weeks. Over time, watch the posterior capsule (behind the IOL) for the appearance of opacity.

If the patient complains of pain postoperatively (beyond the usual), evaluate carefully for corneal abrasion, corneal edema, and intraocular infection.

The eye recovers most of its normal appearance quickly over the first several postoperative days. The remainder of recovery then takes place more slowly over the following weeks.

Retina and Vitreous

Scleral Buckle (Retinal Detachment Repair)

Following retinal detachment repair with a scleral buckle, the patient may have some lid swelling. There may be conjunctival injection, edema, or a subconjunctival hemorrhage. The eye itself is not entered, but there is an incision in the conjunctiva at the limbus. The corneal epithelium may evidence exposure keratitis. Check the AC for inflammatory reaction and hyphema, and monitor chamber depth for angle closure.

One of the risks in retinal detachment repair is the occurrence of anterior segment necrosis, which occurs rarely during the late postoperative course. The slit lamp findings in this complication include marked chemosis; corneal edema; striae; white flakes in the anterior chamber or on the lens; large keratitic precipitates; an irregular, dilated pupil; iris atrophy; posterior synechiae; and cataract formation.

Vitrectomy or Fluid/Gas Exchange

Conjunctival edema, injection, and subconjunctival hemorrhage are normal findings. As with a scleral buckle, the conjunctival incision site is at the limbus. The corneal epithelium may show some punctate staining from exposure. The amount of inflammation in the AC is the most important slit lamp finding. Flare is normal, but cells are generally less visible. The anterior chamber reaction may be quite marked in diabetics. There should not be an hypopyon. Examine the lens for possible cataract formation. (Contact with the lens by the gas markedly increases the chances for cataract development.)

Laser Photocoagulation

While laser photocoagulation is applied to the retina, the slit lamp exam is still vitally important. Mild corneal edema may be present, as well as keratitis from the contact lens used during the procedure. There may also be an anterior chamber reaction. Use transillumination to check for iris atrophy. Note the shape of the pupil. Watch for formation of posterior synechia and cataract.

TABLE 7-1
Postoperative Slit Lamp Examination Notes

I. Lid Surgery

External
Lid swelling
Lid bruising
Lid redness
Skin sloughing
Lid position
Lash position
Presence of a discharge
Broken or missing sutures
Wound gape
Recurrence of lesion(s)
Excessive, irregular scarring (keloids)

Globe
Tearing
Corneal abrasion
Corneal dry spots

II. Lacrimal Surgery

External
Lid swelling
Lid redness
Sutures

Globe
Tearing
Discharge
Silicone tube
Corneal abrasion

III. Enucleation

External
Lid swelling

Socket
Conformer in place
Conjunctival edema (2+ edema would be expected at first)
Conjunctival injection (conjunctiva may look like a piece of raw meat at first)
Presence of conjunctival prolapse (abnormal)
Presence of discharge (a mild mucus discharge is normal)
Sutures

IV. Extraocular Muscles

Globe
Discharge
Injection
Subconjunctival hemorrhage
Conjunctival wound gape
Exposed sutures
Visible choroidal pigment
Corneal abrasion

TABLE 7-1 (continued)
Postoperative Slit Lamp Examination Notes

V. Corneal Transplant

Globe
Wound leak (Seidel's sign)
Ciliary flush
Corneal staining (of any kind)
Corneal edema
Corneal haze
Corneal opacities
Striae
Graft swelling
Rejection line
Vascularization at suture sites
Keratitic precipitates
Broken sutures
Wound leak
Wound dehiscence (gape)
Healing
Anterior chamber reaction
Anterior chamber depth

VI. Pterygium

Globe
Injection
Graft placement
Corneal dry spots
Corneal staining
Corneal edema
Striae
Presence of sutures
AC reaction
Corneal scarring
Presence of new vessels at limbus
Dellen formation

VII. Radial or Astigmatic Keratotomy

Globe
Conjunctival injection
Conjunctival edema
Superficial keratitis
Staining of incision sites
Corneal edema
Corneal infiltrates
Anterior chamber reaction

VIII. Excimer Laser

Globe
Bandage contact lens
    Coverage
    Movement
Re-epithelialization
Flap irregularities (if LASIK)

TABLE 7-1 (continued)
Postoperative Slit Lamp Examination Notes

VIII. Excimer Laser (Continued)

Corneal haze
Corneal infiltrates/inflammation
Recurrent corneal erosion

IX. Surgical Trabeculectomy

Globe
Conjunctival injection
Subconjunctival hemorrhage
Appearance of drainage bleb
Corneal edema
Corneal striae
AC depth
AC reaction
Hyphema
Pupil shape and size
Anterior synechia
Posterior synechia
Cataract formation

X. Laser Trabeculoplasty

Globe
Conjunctival injection
Corneal staining (keratitis most common)
AC reaction
Hyphema
Pupil size and shape
Peripheral anterior synechia

XI. Laser Iridotomy

Globe
Conjunctival injection
Corneal staining (keratitis most common)
AC reaction
Hyphema
Evaluate iridotomy opening
Anterior synechia

XII. Cataract

External
Lid swelling
Ptosis

Globe
Conjunctival injection
Conjunctival chemosis
Wound location
Wound size
Wound gape
Wound leak
Broken sutures

TABLE 7-1 (continued)
Postoperative Slit Lamp Examination Notes

XII. Cataract (Continued)

Globe
Keratitis
Corneal edema
Corneal striae
Endothelial detachment
AC reaction
AC depth
Vitreous in AC
Hyphema
Pupil size
Pupil shape
Location of IOL
Position of IOL
IOL precipitates
Posterior capsule opacity

XIII. Scleral Buckle for Retinal Detachment

External
Lid swelling

Globe
Conjunctival sutures
Conjunctival injection
Conjunctival edema
Subconjunctival hemorrhage
Epithelial staining (exposure keratitis most common)
AC reaction
Hyphema
Cataract

XIV. Vitrectomy or Fluid/Gas Exchange

Globe
Conjunctival sutures
Conjunctival edema
Conjunctival injection
Subconjunctival hemorrhage
Corneal staining/epithelial defects (exposure keratitis most common)
AC reaction
Cataract

XV. Laser Photocoagulation

Globe
Corneal edema
Corneal staining (keratitis most common)
AC reaction
Iris atrophy
Pupil shape
Posterior synechiae
Cataract

Chapter 8

History Mystery

KEY POINTS

- A careful patient history has implications for the entire eye exam.

- Certain patient complaints and symptoms may suggest specific problems that have slit lamp findings.

- Certain slit lamp findings may suggest specific problems with additional slit lamp findings.

- The cause for the patient's subjective visual complaint(s) may be evident on slit lamp examination.

- Subjective physical complaints might be verified with the slit lamp if present at the time of the examination.

Patient symptoms often suggest specific eye problems. When these problems have related slit lamp findings, we can use the patient's complaints to guide the microscopic exam. In this chapter, symptoms are alphabetized and broken into two sections: visual and physical. Under each symptom heading is a list of slit lamp findings that could possibly be related. These are areas you will want to pay close attention to when examining a patient who describes these symptoms. For notes on the appearance and documentation of findings (and, in some cases, actual photographs), see Chapter 5.

Possible ocular causes of physical symptoms are given. However, possible ocular causes of visual symptoms are not investigated; these are either self-explanatory under the description of the slit lamp exam or are not evident with the slit lamp (such as retinal disorders). Possible systemic causes are listed in both sections, when appropriate (some are admittedly rare). These include diseases and conditions as well as allergic and drug reactions. If your patient reports symptoms that do not seem to have slit lamp related causes, explore the possibility of systemic origins. Then, refer to Chapter 6 for other slit lamp findings related to specific conditions and drugs. It is often a particular combination of findings that leads the physician to a diagnosis.

Note: Most of the material in this chapter has been adapted with permission from *The Crystal Clear Guide to Sight for Life*, Starburst Publishers, 1996.

Visual Symptoms

• **Blurry vision**

Slit lamp exam: coated contact lens, poorly aligned astigmatic or bifocal contact lens, contact lens induced corneal problems, closed angles, foreign matter in tear film, corneal opacities, corneal edema, corneal guttata, keratitis (toxic or infectious), cloudy aqueous, cycloplegia/mydriasis, lens opacities, dislocated lens, capsule opacity, dislocated IOL

Possible systemic causes: diabetes, poorly controlled blood pressure, drug reaction, vitamin deficiency, hormonal disorders, arteriosclerosis

• **Color vision, change in**

Slit lamp exam: cataract

Possible systemic causes: drug toxicity

• **Distorted vision**

Slit lamp exam: poorly aligned toric contact lens, corneal irregularities, keratoconus, lens opacities

• **Double vision**

Slit lamp exam: foreign matter in tear film, poorly aligned toric contact lens, poorly centered contact lens, corneal irregularities, lens opacities, dislocated lens, dislocated IOL, capsule opacity

Possible systemic causes: stroke, multiple sclerosis, thyroid trouble, diabetes, vitamin toxicity, nerve palsy

• **Fluctuating vision**

Slit lamp exam: chalazion (due to pressure on cornea), foreign matter in tear film, contact lens too tight or too loose, contact lens not moving properly, corneal guttata, corneal edema, keratoconus, prior corneal refractive surgery, dry eye, lens opacities

Possible systemic cause: diabetes

• **Glare**

Slit lamp exam: poorly aligned toric or bifocal contact lens, poorly centered contact lens, corneal scar or other opacities, corneal dystrophy, keratoconus, lens opacities, capsule opacity, dislocated IOL

Possible systemic cause: drug reaction

• **Halos around lights at night**

Slit lamp exam: tight contact lens, mucus on cornea, corneal scar, corneal edema, closed or narrow angles, lens opacities, dislocated IOL, capsule opacity

Possible systemic cause: drug reaction

• **Improvement of near vision**

Slit lamp exam: nuclear sclerosis

Possible systemic cause: diabetes

• **Loss of depth perception**

Slit lamp exam: corneal opacities, lens opacities, capsule opacity

• **Loss of near vision**

Slit lamp exam: lens opacities, capsule opacity

Possible systemic cause: drug reaction

• **Loss of upper vision**

Slit lamp exam: ptosis, dermatochalasis

• **Loss of vision (gradual)**

Slit lamp exam: contact lens deposits, corneal dystrophy, lens opacities, capsule opacity

Possible systemic causes: diabetes, vitamin toxicity, drug reaction

• **Loss of vision (sudden)**

Slit lamp exam: closed angles (with resultant corneal edema)

Possible systemic causes: drug reaction, temporal arteritis, stroke, multiple sclerosis, tumor exerting pressure on optic tract

• **Moving vision (vision seems to vibrate)**

Slit lamp exam: nystagmus

Possible systemic causes: alcoholism, CNS damage, endocarditis, Marfan's Syndrome, multiple sclerosis

• **Poor night vision**

Slit lamp exam: corneal dystrophy, lens opacities, capsule opacity

Possible systemic cause: Vitamin A deficiency

• **Uncomfortable vision**

Slit lamp exam: contact lens too tight, poor or absent blinking, conjunctival dryness, poor tear film, excessive tearing, corneal dryness, exposure keratitis

Physical Symptoms

• **Aching eye**

Slit lamp exam: lid lesions, episcleral/scleral nodule, conjunctival injection, corneal edema, keratitic precipitates, cell and flare, narrow or closed angles, anisocoria, decreased tear film

Possible ocular causes: angle closure glaucoma, iritis, episcleritis, scleritis, trauma, dry eye

Possible systemic causes: gout, lupus, rheumatoid arthritis, Herpes zoster (shingles), sinus infection, sarcoid

• **Burning**

Slit lamp exam: check tear film, conjunctival dryness, and corneal integrity; conjunctival injection

Possible ocular causes: dry eye, allergy, chemical burn (including contact lens solutions)

Possible systemic cause: drug reaction

• **Crusting lids**

Possible concurrent slit lamp findings: lid swelling, lice/nits in lashes, lash loss, rash, oozing

Possible ocular causes: blepharitis, contact allergy (including topical medications), eczema

Possible systemic causes: psoriasis, rosacea, seborrheic dermatitis

• **Difference in pupil size (anisocoria)**

Possible concurrent slit lamp findings: corneal edema, cell and flare in aqueous, closed angles, keratitic precipitates

Possible ocular causes: angle closure glaucoma, surgery, trauma, iritis, accidental dilation, reaction to topical medications, Horner's syndrome

Possible systemic causes: congenital, head trauma, chemical exposure

• **Foreign body sensation (grittiness)**

Slit lamp exam: check cleanliness of contact lens, check tear film, check lid and lash position; rash, hordeolum, chalazion, lice/nits in lashes, conjunctival injection, conjunctival chemosis, conjunctival dryness, conjunctival concretions, papillae, episcleral nodule, broken or exposed sutures, corneal dryness, keratitis, foreign body

Possible ocular causes: foreign body (loose, conjunctival, corneal), conjunctivitis, sutures, corneal abrasion, keratitis, corneal ulcer or dendrite, corneal laceration, dry eye, trichiasis, entropion, ectropion, conjunctival calcifications, deposits on contact lens, ultraviolet burn, chemical burn (including contact lens solutions), allergic reaction to topical medications, other allergies (including waste products of lice), thermal burn, incomplete lid closure, growth or lesion on lid, recurrent corneal erosion, inflamed pinguecula, giant papillary conjunctivitis

Possible systemic causes: drug reaction, Herpes simplex, Bell's palsy, psoriasis, rheumatoid arthritis

• **Growths (See Table 5-1)**

Possible slit lamp findings: mole, xanthelasma, hordeolum, chalazion, cancer, wart, cyst, skin tag

Possible systemic causes: AIDS (Kaposi's sarcoma), allergic reaction, measles (Koplik's spot), neurofibromatosis (Von Recklinghausen's Disease), elevated cholesterol (xanthelasma)

• **Headaches**

Slit lamp exam: lid lesions, dermatochalasis, limbal injection, corneal edema, narrow or closed angles

Possible ocular causes: dermatochalasis (from strain of holding brows up in order to elevate lids), angle closure glaucoma, drug reaction

Possible systemic causes: Herpes zoster, high blood pressure, drug reaction, carotid artery disease, temporal arteritis

Note: There are obviously many more systemic causes of headaches. We have only listed those with other potential slit lamp findings.

- **Itching**

    Slit lamp exam: lid rash, lash crusting, lid swelling, oozing lid lesions, lice/nits in lashes, lash loss, follicles, papillae, conjunctival injection, conjunctival chemosis

    Possible ocular causes: blepharitis, allergies, drug reaction, contact allergy (including topical medications and contact lens solutions), eczema

    Possible systemic cause: drug reaction

- **Jumping eyelid**

    Possible concurrent slit lamp findings: corneal or conjunctival injury

    Possible ocular causes: pain, injury

    Possible systemic causes: Parkinson's disease, caffeine, drug reaction, stress, lack of sleep, underactive parathyroid, lack of calcium

- **Lash loss**

    Possible concurrent slit lamp findings: lash crusting, lid redness and/or swelling

    Possible ocular causes: blepharitis

    Possible systemic causes: leprosy, thyroid (underactive), psychosis, seborrheic dermatitis

- **Lid droop**

    Possible concurrent slit lamp findings: injury, growths

    Possible ocular causes: ptosis, dermatochalasis, growths, injury

    Possible systemic causes: muscular dystrophy, myasthenia gravis, 3rd nerve palsy, neurofibromatosis

- **Lid swelling**

    Possible concurrent slit lamp findings: lid redness, rash, crusting lashes, oozing, injury

    Possible ocular causes: infection (cellulitis, blepharitis, hordeolum, chalazion), injury, allergic reaction to topical medication or chemicals (including contact lens solutions)

    Possible systemic causes: malnutrition, mononucleosis, Herpes zoster, overactive thyroid, underactive thyroid, drug reaction, fluid retention, malnutrition

- **Light sensitivity (*see also Glare*)**

    Slit lamp exam: broken corneal integrity, cell and flare, pupil size and reaction, absence of iris

    Possible ocular causes: dilation, drug reaction, iritis, corneal injury or infection, aniridia

    Possible systemic causes: systemic inflammatory disease, albinism

- **Matter/discharge**

    Possible concurrent slit lamp findings: conjunctival injection, conjunctival chemosis, follicles, papillae, keratitis

    Possible ocular causes: infection, allergy

- **Pain**

    See Aching eye or Foreign body sensation

- **Protrusion of the eye(s)**

    Possible concurrent slit lamp findings: abnormal lid position, conjunctival dryness, exposure keratitis

    Possible ocular causes: unilateral ptosis (drooped lid makes it appear as though opposite eye is protruding), orbital tumor

    Possible systemic causes: Graves' Disease (overactive thyroid), drug or vitamin toxicity

- **Rash**

    Possible concurrent slit lamp findings: lid erythema, lid edema, oozing, lash crusting

    Possible ocular causes: allergic reaction to drugs or chemicals (including contact lens solutions), contact dermatitis

    Possible systemic causes: chickenpox, Herpes zoster (shingles), Herpes simplex, lupus, small pox, vaccinia, eczema

- **Redness**

    Possible concurrent slit lamp findings: rash, lice in lashes, lash crusting, conjunctival edema, conjunctival dryness, papillae, episcleral nodule, discharge, poor tear film, little or no movement of contact lens, deposits on contact lens, corneal edema, corneal erosion or other breaks, keratitic precipitates, cell and flare, narrow or closed angles, mid dilated pupil, miosis

    Possible ocular causes: angle closure glaucoma, dry eye, iritis, conjunctivitis, keratitis, episcleritis, scleritis, injury, subconjunctival hemorrhage, chemical reaction (including contact lens solutions), allergic reaction to topical medications, allergic reaction to waste products of lice, inflamed pinguecula, inflamed pterygium, tight contact lens, giant papillary conjunctivitis, dirty contact lens

    Possible systemic causes: drug reaction, inflammatory diseases (carotid artery disease, gout, rheumatoid arthritis, etc), hay fever, asthma, eczema

    Possible systemic causes of subconjunctival hemorrhage: hypertension, anemia, drug reaction (blood thinners), Vitamin C deficiency, straining

- **Watery eyes**

    Slit lamp exam: check tear lake, tear film, and lid position; poor tear film, incomplete lid closure, poor or absent blink, conjunctival dryness, conjunctival injection, conjunctival or corneal foreign body, corneal dryness, keratitis, exposure keratitis, corneal injury

    Possible ocular causes: dry eye, foreign body, injury, allergy, drug reaction, infection, trichiasis, entropion, ectropion

    Possible external causes: smoke, fumes, moving/blowing air, low humidity

Chapter 9

Contact Lens Evaluation for Nonfitters

KEY POINTS

- The slit lamp exam is key in determining candidacy for contact lenses.

- Regular fluorescein dye will stain soft contact lenses!

- A lens that is placed on the eye in the office should be allowed at least 30 minutes to equilibrate.

- The slit lamp exam is used to differentiate between blurred vision caused by the contact lens vs. that caused by corneal compromise.

- The contact lens patient must be examined with the lenses both on and off.

- Some slit lamps have a lens holder attachment for evaluation of soft or rigid lenses. This makes it possible to evaluate the lens surface without the interference of secretions, blinks, and tears.

Slit Lamp Exam of the Prospective Contact Lens Patient

The result of the slit lamp examination is one of the determining factors in whether or not a patient can try contact lenses. Here is a basic list of things that the fitter will want to know:

1. Tear film: Is the tear film clear, or is there evidence of oil and/or debris? What is the tear BUT? Is there evidence of dry eye?

2. Eyelids: What is the blink rate? Do the lids close completely with each blink? Are the lid margins smooth? Is exophthalmus present? Are the lids and lashes clean, or is there crusting and evidence of infection? How does the female patient wear eye makeup (heavy mascara, liner on the lid margins, etc)?

3. Conjunctiva: Is there any redness? (If yes, give location and grade.) Are there any growths that might interfere with the location of a contact lens? Are there any papillae or follicles on the palpebral conjunctiva?

4. Cornea: Is the cornea totally clear? Are there any scars? Dystrophy? Vascularization? When fluorescein dye is applied, is there any staining?

Slit Lamp Exam of the Soft Contact Lens (Table 9-1)

Hygiene

One of the first things you will notice about a soft contact lens is its surface. Build up of film and deposits generally (but not always) indicate how well the patient is complying with cleaning regimens. A soft lens may become filmed over with mucus secretion from the eye itself. This is especially common in lenses worn on an extended basis. Deposits are material that have precipitated out of the tear film and adhered to the lens (Figure 9-1). Calcium (mineral) deposits look like grains of salt. "Jelly bumps" are smooth, round, white, glistening deposits that are a combination of lipid and calcium. Protein may appear as a diffuse haze with poor wetting over the deposits. Note the appearance and degree of any deposits or films, rating from 0+ to 4+. (Examples: hygiene- fair; 3+ jelly bumps; 2+ film.)

You should also note the tear film. Is there oil, debris, or makeup in the tears? Do the tears swab evenly over the lens surface, or are there spots where the tears break up on the lens?

Coverage, Movement, and Centration

First, compare the diameter of the lens to the diameter of the cornea. Does the lens edge cover the entire cornea and extend onto the limbus? Does the lens touch the limbus in any area? Is any part of the cornea not covered by the lens (ie, exposed)? A soft lens should overlap the limbus by 1.0 mm on all sides (Figure 9-2). Areas that are not covered tend to dry out, and may stain with fluorescein. In addition, chronic redness may develop adjacent to the exposed area. In extreme cases a dellen (a shallow excavated area) may form. Note the location of the lens edges in the patient's chart. (Examples: covers well; inferior nasal exposed.)

A lens of standard thickness should move 0.50 to 1.00 mm with every blink and on upgaze. Less movement may be seen in an ultrathin lens (0.50 mm). Movement more than 1.00 mm may indicate a loose lens. A bandage lens may be fit with little or no movement if the corneal

TABLE 9-1
Soft Contact Lens Evaluation

- **hygiene/cleanliness:** look for deposits, film.
Doc: note, describe, grade 1+ to 4+

- **coverage:** generally, a soft contact lens will extend beyond the limbus in every direction; the edge will not be on the cornea.
Doc: note, describe ("limbal touch nasally," etc)

- **movement:** a soft lens will generally move about 1.00 mm with a blink. If it does not, have the patient look up; you should see a 1.00 mm downward slide of the lens. If it still does not move, have the patient blink while looking up; there should now be 1.00 mm movement.
Doc: note ("good," "excessive," "none," etc)

- **centration:** ideally the optical center of the lens will align with the patient's visual axis. If the lens is offcenter, this should be noted.
Doc: describe ("good," "centers temporally," etc)

- **alignment:** an astigmatic lens has marks to evaluate lens alignment.
Doc: describe location of mark(s) as if the eye were a clock ("astig rides at 6:00," "astig rides at 7:00," etc)

- **integrity:** look for tears, holes, etc.
Doc: note, give location of any defect, if possible ("edge," "center," etc)

- **corneal staining:** the healthy cornea will not stain. Stain indicates a broken epithelial layer.
Doc: note, draw, or describe giving location and extent ("cornea clear," "3+ central staining," etc)

- **other:** look for bubbles, puckers, anything else unusual.
Doc: note, describe

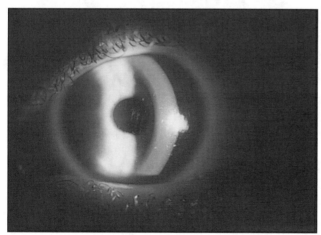

Figure 9-1. Deposits on a soft contact lens (visible in the beam). (Photo by Val Sanders.)

Figure 9-2. A well fit soft lens covers the entire limbus. (Photo by Patrick Caroline.)

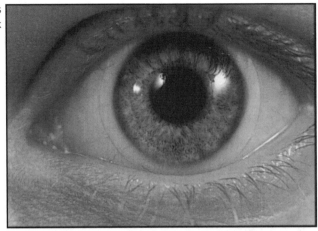

Figure 9-3. Soft lens drifts off cornea in upgaze. (Photo courtesy Bausch and Lomb.)

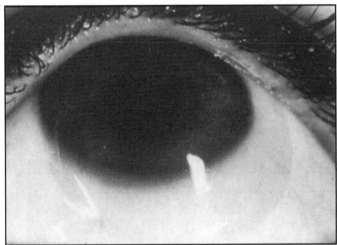

epithelium is broken. If the corneal surface is intact, movement of 0.50 to 1.00 mm is acceptable in a bandage lens. If you cannot see any movement when the patient blinks in primary gaze, have him or her blink while looking up. Also, have the patient look left and right, watching how the lens follows the eye. If movement is adequate, the lens will lag 0.50 to 1.00 mm in the lateral gazes. When you document notes on lens movement, simply describe what you see. (Examples: adequate movement; moves only on upgaze; no movement.)

Note where the lens settles after the blink (Figures 9-3 and 9-4). Ideally, the optical center of the lens should be in line with the patient's visual axis. A lens may be large enough to cover the entire cornea and overlap onto the limbus, yet may center so that a portion of the cornea is left exposed. Describe the off-center location by giving the direction of decentration. (Example: decentered nasally.) In addition, a lens may decenter during the blink and drift back into place after the blink. Make a note of this, as well. (Example: decenters vertically with blink.)

Lens centration is of critical importance when fitting soft astigmatic lenses. Typically, these lenses are marked with dots or lines to aid in evaluation (Figure 9-5). Depending on the type of lens, the mark should ride at 6:00, or on the horizontal meridian (Figure 9-6). Have the patient blink while you watch the mark. Does it return to the same position after each blink? Is it properly aligned? Report the alignment of the mark by describing it as if the eye were a clock

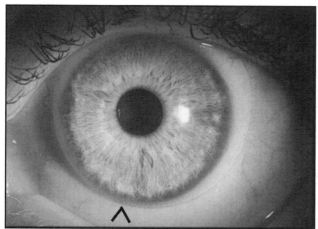

Figure 9-4. Soft lens decentration, with limbal touch inferiorly at caret. (Photo by Patrick Caroline.)

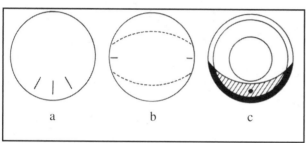

a   b   c

Figure 9-5. Markings on toric contact lenses.

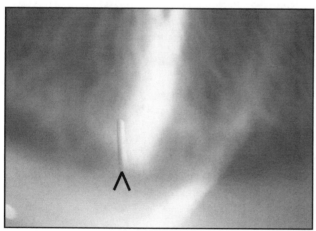

Figure 9-6. Correctly aligned soft toric lens, with mark falling at 6:00. (Photo by Patrick Caroline.)

(example: mark rides at 7:00). Some slit lamps have an angle scale built into the ocular. Otherwise, you might rotate the slit (not possible on all models) to match the mark on the lens by turning the instrument's slit rotation control ring. The angle of the rotation is indicated on a scale. If the astigmatic lens is centered by truncation (the bottom of the lens is flattened off), examine its position. It is important to note, however, that the truncation may not be a guide to the cylinder axis because the lower lid may be sloped.

Alignment is also key in bifocal contacts. These lenses may also be truncated (flattened on the bottom edge) or prism ballasted (thicker on the bottom edge for weight) to assist in positioning.

Lens Characteristics

Signs of a Tight Lens

There are several slit lamp findings that may indicate that a lens is too tight. There may be redness at the corneal/limbal junction for 360 degrees. When the patient blinks, the lens may appear to move when, in fact, it is really pulling the conjunctiva. (Look at the tiny conjunctival vessels at the lens' edge and ask the patient to blink. If the fit is tight, the lens will pull on the vessels, known as conjunctival drag.) Bubbles may be trapped under the tight lens, as well. When the patient removes the tight lens, you may see corneal haze as well as an indentation mark on the sclera indicating where the lens touched.

Signs of a Loose Lens

A loose lens may drop more than 1.00 mm when the patient looks up. If the patient looks to the right or left, the lens may stay in the center instead of following the eye (lens lag). A loose lens may ride high or temporally. The edges may be puckered or stand out from the surface of the eye. This later situation, known as edge lift or standoff, can also occur if the lens is inverted (inside out).

 ## Associated Problems

Corneal Hypoxia

Hypoxia is the condition of low oxygen (*hypo-*, meaning low, and *-oxia*, referring to oxygen). Oxygen supply to the cornea is critical in contact lens wear, particularly with soft contacts. Slit lamp findings of the hypoxic cornea can include neovascularization (especially in the superior quadrant), generalized corneal edema (best viewed with sclerotic scatter), edematous corneal formations (ECF), vertical striae, and corneal infiltrates. These findings are noted in the patient's chart and graded subjectively.

Giant Papillary Conjunctivitis

You should always check the palpebral conjunctiva of the soft contact lens wearer. The appearance of large papillae (particularly under the upper lid) and copious mucous discharge indicate giant papillary conjunctivitis (GPC). This is probably due to a reaction to protein deposits on the lens, so double check lens hygiene, as well. You may subjectively grade GPC using numbers 1+ to 4+ or written description (such as "moderate" and "severe").

Corneal Infections

The soft contact lens can act as a carrier for bacteria and protozoa. Such contamination is much more likely in a dirty lens, as the protein deposits provide food for the organisms. In extended lens wear, the sleeping eye provides a warm, moist, low-oxygenated environment in which some bacteria thrive. The cornea of a contact lens wearer (particularly if he or she is complaining of redness, discomfort, and/or discharge) should be evaluated carefully at each visit. For documentation you may want to draw a picture or write a description indicating the location and number of infiltrates.

TABLE 9-2
Rigid Contact Lens Evaluation

- **hygiene/cleanliness:** look for deposits, film.
Doc: note, grade 1+ to 4+, describe.

- **ride/centration:** ideally, the center of the lens should come to rest over the optic zone of the pupil.
Doc: note, describe decentration ("nasal ride," "superior ride," etc).

- **movement:** a rigid lens will usually be drawn up by a blink, then slide down into place right after the blink.
Doc: describe ("good," "excessive," "none," etc) or grade 1+ to 4+.

- **fluorescein dye pattern:** a properly fit lens will generally have a thin, even layer of dye under it with slight pooling in the periphery.
Doc: describe ("good dye pattern," "pooling under central lens," etc).

- **lens surface:** an even coat of tears should be swabbed over the lens with every blink.
Doc: describe ("good wetting," "several dry spots," "poor wetting").

- **integrity:** look for chips, crazing, scratches.
Doc: note, describe, grade scratches 1+ to 4+.

- **bifocal segments:** alignment is critical with these lenses.
Doc: describe ("seg well aligned," "lower seg rocks temporally," etc).

- **corneal staining:** the healthy cornea will not stain. Stain indicates a broken epithelial layer.
Doc: note, draw, or describe location and extent ("cornea clear," "3+ central staining," etc).

- **bubbles under lens:** in the average fit, there should not be any bubbles under the lens.
Doc: note location.

Corneal Staining

First, remember that ordinary fluorescein dye will stain a soft contact lens. If you accidentally put the dye into an eye with a soft lens, remove and irrigate the lens immediately with sterile saline. Then clean the lens with the patient's habitual cleaner. Fluoresoft™, however, may be safely instilled with a soft lens in place.

Corneal staining in the soft lens wearer is usually due to mechanical irritation or solution sensitivity. However, it may also be associated with corneal infections as mentioned above and manifested as punctate keratitis or ulcers. Corneal abrasions can occur with soft lenses as well, most notably with incorrect insertion and removal techniques. Sensitivity to chemicals used in cleaning the lenses may cause a diffuse keratitis. A drawing or written description and grading of the staining should be noted in the patient's record. (Examples: 4+ diffuse staining; 2+ central staining; 2.00 mm stained area inferior nasal.)

Slit Lamp Exam of the Rigid Contact Lens (Table 9-2)

Hygiene

Like soft lenses, rigid lenses can also be plagued by deposits. Because of the lens material, these deposits may be manifest more as a waxy coating on the lens. It is easier to see this if you

Figure 9-7. Alignment fit gas permeable lens. This example shows a well-fit lens. (Photo by Patrick Caroline, courtesy Bausch and Lomb/Polymer Technology.)

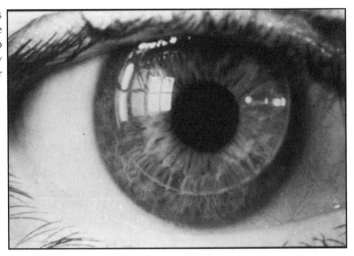

Figure 9-8. Lens adhesion. Note nasal decentration and debris trapped under lens. (Photo by Patrick Caroline, courtesy Bausch and Lomb/Polymer Technology.)

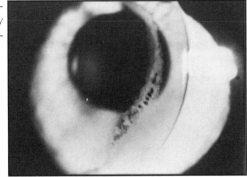

remove the lens, then rinse and dry it before holding it up to the slit lamp. Describe any deposits or coatings, and grade their presence from 0+ to 4+. (Examples: good hygiene; 2+ waxy deposits.)

Movement and Centration

A rigid lens is smaller than a soft lens and, thus, will not cover the cornea. The old PMMA hard contact lenses were designed to have an interpalpebral fit. That is, the centered lens lies entirely between the lids. The more modern method of fitting gas permeable lenses (which are larger than PMMA contacts) is the alignment fit, where the upper third of the lens stays under the upper lid (Figure 9-7).

The movement of a rigid lens is much different from that of a soft lens. The rigid lens will move slightly upward with each blink (about 1.00 to 2.00 mm), then smoothly drift down and resettle. It should not "drop" down. Normally, the lens should not bump into the lower lid margin. When the patient looks left or right, the contact may lag 0.50 to 1.00 mm behind, but it should not move past the limbus. Adhesion of the lens to the cornea (usually in a decentered position) is a common occurrence (Figure 9-8). Movement is noted and described in the chart. (Examples: adequate movement; lens falls to lower lid after blink.)

Ideally, the lens will center so that the optical zone of the contact falls in front of the patient's visual axis. Make a note if you see that the lens is riding high (Figure 9-9A), low (Figure 9-9B), or laterally.

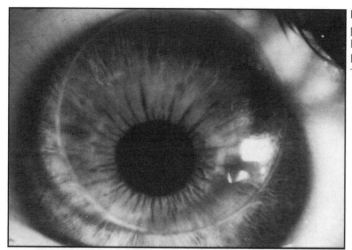

Figure 9-9A. High-riding gas permeable lens. (Photo by Patrick Caroline, courtesy Bausch and Lomb/Polymer Technology.)

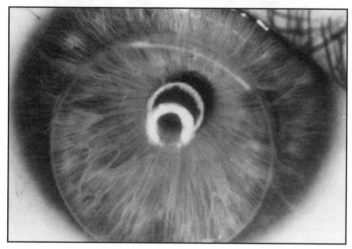

Figure 9-9B. Low-riding gas permeable lens. (Photo by Patrick Caroline, courtesy Bausch and Lomb/Polymer Technology.)

Rigid lenses can be left in place when fluorescein dye is instilled. In fact, observing the pattern of the dye under and around the lens provides the fitter with valuable information about the lens fit. If you, as a nonfitter, are asked to evaluate the fluorescein pattern, the general rule is to note areas where the dye pools and areas where the dye is absent. Be sure to use the cobalt blue filter. The appearance of the dye may be further enhanced by the use of a #12 (yellow) Wrattan filter. The Wrattan filter blocks out excess blue light, thus enhancing the green color of the dye. The background becomes dark. The filter is available at photography/camera shops. To use the filter with the slit lamp, hold or tape it on the patient side of the instrument.

If the fluorescein reflex is bright green and the tear layer is thick, there is clearance between the contact lens and the cornea. A faint green reflex and a thin tear layer indicate minimum clearance. If the reflex appears black and there is no tear layer, then the lens is touching the cornea. In a good fit, a thin film of dye will be evenly spread under the entire lens, with slight pooling at the periphery. If the patient has astigmatism, you might see a band of dye running horizontally or vertically. A loose (flat) lens will show a central absence of dye and a pooling around the edge (Figure 9-10). A tight (steep) lens will have pooling in the center and an absence of dye at the periphery (Figure 9-11). (There are exceptions.) For documentation, simply draw or describe what you see.

Figure 9-10. A loose (flat) gas permeable lens with pooling at lens edges. (Photo by Val Sanders.)

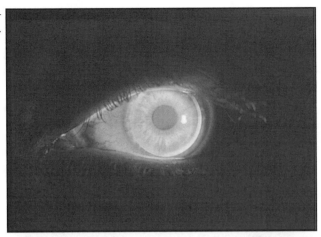

Figure 9-11. A tight (steep) gas permeable lens with no dye at lens edges. (Photo by Val Sanders.)

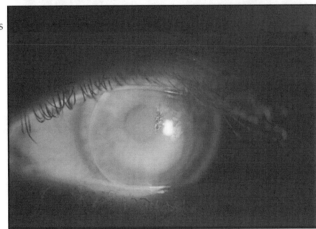

Lens Appearance

Each time the patient blinks, a smooth sheet of tears should be swabbed over the lens. This may be best observed after fluorescein dye has been instilled. If the tears bead up on the lens or dry spots appear immediately after the blink, note this in the record.

Lens clouding may have several causes. If the lens surface is not smooth, the eye may respond with an increase in mucus or oily discharge. This occurs regardless of lens hygiene. Lenses may also cloud if the patient is mixing incompatible cleaning chemicals. Processes used in lens manufacture can also cause haziness. You can subjectively grade lens clouding using 1+ to 4+. (Examples: lens clear; 3+ lens clouding.)

The surface of a rigid lens may become crazed. (Have you ever seen an old china plate where the finish on the plate had a network of tiny cracks all over it? That is crazing.) In a contact lens, this can be caused by a plaque on the lens that interferes with wetting and should be noted in the chart.

Carefully examine the edges of the lens for chips and nicks and note them in the record. (The bottom of the lens may be purposely flattened or truncated to provide for better lens stability.) Check the lens surface for cracks and scratches. Scratches may be subjectively graded from 0+ to 4+.

The segments of a fused or one-piece rigid bifocal contact lens will be visible with the slit lamp. Note where the segment line falls when the lens recenters after a blink.

Associated Problems

Corneal Hypoxia

OptA

Corneal hypoxia (lack of oxygen) in rigid lenses often causes an area of edema that is central, rather than diffuse as in soft lenses. This central area is round or oval (in the case of astigmatism), about 2.00 to 4.00 mm across, and grayish white. Draw or describe and grade any edema that is present. The edema becomes more dense as the condition worsens and may eventually be visible without the slit lamp. The problem may also be accompanied by superficial punctate corneal staining (see Corneal Staining below).

Corneal Infiltrates

Corneal infiltrates are congregations of white blood cells and lymphocytes that form in response to a viral infection, chemical sensitivity, or lack of oxygen. They look like little dots under the epithelium and may be surrounded by a tiny fuzzy border of edema. You may draw or describe them.

Corneal Staining

Our concern here is the corneal staining patterns that present when the lens has been removed. Consult Figure 9-12 and use it to draw or describe any corneal staining that you observe. In addition to the patterns shown, another possible cause of staining is a phenomenon known as dimple veiling (Figure 9-13). In this situation, bubbles form under the lens. The bubbles put pressure on the cornea and cause tiny depressions in the corneal epithelium. These depressions, which usually occur centrally or superiorly, will stain with the dye.

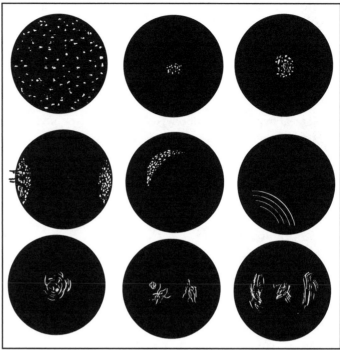

Figure 9-12. Common types of rigid lens staining. Top left: Diffuse punctate staining. Usually chemical or environmental in origin. Often related to solution sensitivity. Top center: Apical staining. Often due to poor lens/cornea relationship. Common in keratoconus patients. Top right: Overwear stain (epithelial erosion). Middle left: 3:00 and 9:00 staining. Attributed to lid gap, poor blink pattern, mechanical trauma. Desiccation occurs in areas adjacent to lens edge at approximately 3:00 and 9:00. Middle center: Arcuate stain. Usually due to edge defect, poor edge design, or dried mucus on lens. Middle right: Recentering stain. Can also occur from faulty insertion technique. Bottom left: Swirl-like stain. Seen with poor lens/cornea relationship and in keratoconus patients with apical touch. Bottom center: Foreign body stain. Bottom right: Mucus deposits or scratched lens stain. (Adapted with permission from Koch et al. *Adverse Effects of Contact Lens Wear.* SLACK Incorporated.)

Figure 9-13. Dimple veiling. Note collection of small bubbles under lens. (Photo courtesy Bausch and Lomb/Polymer Technology.)

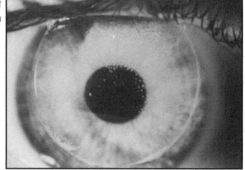

References

References

Benes SC, McKinney K, Sanders LC, Miller MG, Moberg M. *Advanced Ophthalmic Diagnostics and Therapeutics.* Thorofare, NJ: SLACK Incorporated; 1992.

Berkow R, ed. *The Merck Manual.* 15th ed. Rahway, NJ: Merck Sharp & Dohme Research Laboratories; 1987.

Borover BB, Langley TS. *Office and Career Management for the Eyecare Paraprofessional.* Thorofare, NJ: SLACK Incorporated; 1997.

Cassin B. *Fundamentals for Ophthalmic Technical Personnel.* Philadelphia, Pa: WB Saunders; 1995.

Cogger TJ. Correction with hard contact lenses. In: Duane TD, ed. *Clinical Ophthalmology.* Philadelphia, Pa: Harper and Row; 1984.

Craig CR, Stitzel RE, eds. *Modern Pharmacology.* 3rd ed. Boston, Mass: Little, Brown and Company; 1990.

Cunningham D. *Clinical Ocular Photography.* Thorofare, NJ: SLACK Incorporated; 1998.

Cutina A. Adaptation of the slit lamp for patients with large breasts [letter]. *Ophthalmic Surg.* 1991;22(10):623.

Dewart M. Basic slit lamp techniques. *Eye Quest Magazine.* 1992;2(2):16,18-19,21,23-24.

Gayton JL, Kershner R. *Refractive Surgery for Eyecare Paraprofessionals.* Thorofare, NJ: SLACK Incorporated; 1997.

Gayton JL, Ledford JK. *The Crystal Clear Guide to Sight for Life.* Lancaster, Pa: Starburst Publishers; 1996.

Gean CJ, Hiatt GFS, Meyers FH. *Pocket Drug Guide.* Baltimore, Md: Williams and Wilkins; 1989.

Herrin MP. *Ophthalmic Examination and Basic Skills.* Thorofare, NJ: SLACK Incorporated; 1990.

Josephson JE, Caffery BE. Corneal staining after installation of topical anesthetic. *Investigative Ophthalmology and Visual Science.* 1988;29:1096-1099.

Kershner R, Duvall B. *Ophthalmic Medications and Pharmacology.* 2nd ed. Thorofare, NJ: SLACK Incorporated; 2005.

Luntz MH. Clinical types of cataract. In: Duane TD, ed. *Clinical Ophthalmology.* Philadelphia, Pa: Harper and Row; 1984.

Nemeth SC, Shea CA. *Medical Sciences for the Ophthalmic Assistant.* Thorofare, NJ: SLACK Incorporated; 1988.

Pavan-Langston D, ed. *Manual of Ocular Diagnosis and Therapy.* 2nd ed. Boston, Mass: Little, Brown and Company; 1985.

Phelps CD. Examination and functional evaluation of the crystalline lens. In: Duane TD, ed. *Clinical Ophthalmology.* Philadelphia, Pa: Harper and Row; 1984.

Physician's Desk Reference. 58th ed. on CD-ROM. Montvale, NJ: Thomson PDR; 2004.

Pickett K. *Overview of Ocular Surgery, and Surgical Counseling.* Thorofare, NJ: SLACK Incorporated; 1999.

Premarket Notification (510[k]) Guidance Document for Daily Wear Contact Lenses. Rockville, Md: US Food and Drug Administration; 1994.

Rakow PL. *Contact Lenses.* Thorofare, NJ: SLACK Incorporated; 1988.

Rakow PL. Evaluating the lens fit. *Vision Care Assistant.* 1991; Jan/Feb:8.

Rose WE Jr. Documentation: boon or bane, part 2. *Ocular Surgery News.* 1991;6(17):23.

Scott WE, D'Agostino DD, Lennarson LW. *Orthoptics and Ocular Examination Techniques.* Baltimore, Md: Williams and Wilkins; 1983.

Spaeth GL, ed. *Ophthalmic Surgery: Principles and Practice.* Philadelphia, Pa: WB Saunders; 1982.

Stein HA, Cheskes A, Stein RM. *The Excimer: Fundamentals and Clinical Use.* Thorofare, NJ: SLACK Incorporated; 1995.

Stein HA, Slatt BJ. *Fitting Guide for Rigid and Soft Contact Lenses.* 2nd ed. St Louis, Mo: Mosby; 1984.

Stein HA, Slatt BJ, Stein RM. *The Ophthalmic Assistant.* 6th ed. St Louis, Mo: Mosby; 1994.

Tasman W. The vitreous. In: Duane TD, ed. *Clinical Ophthalmology.* Philadelphia, Pa: Harper and Row; 1984.

US Food and Drug Administration website: http://www.accessdata.fda.gov/scripts/cder/drugsatfda/index.cfm?fuseaction=Search.Search_Drug_Name; Accessed 6/16/05.

Vaughan DG, Asbury T, Riordan-Eva P. *General Ophthalmology.* 13th ed. Norwalk, Conn: Appleton and Lange; 1992.

Waring GO, Laibson PR. A systematic method of drawing corneal pathologic conditions. *Archives of Ophthalmology.* 1977;95:1540-1542.

Index

abbreviations, for documentation, 20, 31
abrasions, corneal, 67, 72, 89
    in contact lens wear, 129
    postoperative, 104, 105, 111, 113
abscess, postoperative, 108
abuse, physical, 89
acne, 89
acquired immunodeficiency syndrome (AIDS), 89
albinism, 89
alcoholism, 89
alignment
    of contact lenses, 125, 126-127, 129-130
    of patient, 14
allergy, 89, 104
anatomical directions, 30
anemia, 89
angle(s)
    examination of, 6, 22, 40-41, 53
    grading of, 75-76
angle closure glaucoma, 41
angle opening, 75
angle scale, 2, 127
angle scale index, 2
anisocoria, 120
ankylosing spondylitis, 89
anterior chamber
    depth of, 41, 114, 115
    examination of, 2, 22, 27, 40-42
    findings in, 75-76
    intraocular lens in, 42
    postoperative, 105-106, 110, 111, 112, 114, 115, 116
anterior segment, examination of, 40-44
anterior uveitis, 87
anterior vitreous face, 44
aqueous, 40-41, 49, 106
arcus senilis, 67
arteriosclerosis, 89
A-scan ultrasound, 6
asteroid hyalosis, 84
asthma, 90
astigmatic keratectomy, 107
astigmatism, 107-109, 126, 133
atrophy, iris, 77, 112, 116

band keratopathy, 67
bandage contact lens, 109, 114, 124, 126
basal cell carcinoma, 61
beam, 46. *See also* slit beam
Bell's palsy, 90
bifocal contact lenses, 127, 129, 133
biomicroscope, 2
black eye, 88
bleb, monitoring, 109-110, 115
blepharitis, 31, 86
blepharospasm, 59
blink(ing)
    in contact lens wear, 124, 126, 128, 130, 132
    evaluation of, 37
    tear film and, 37-38
blood vessels. *See also* neovascularization, corneal
    abnormal, in cornea, 106
    episclera, 38
    ghost, 68
    iris, 42-43, 78
    leash, 64
    at limbus, 38
blue filters, 20
Bowman's membrane, 39-40
breakup time, tear (BUT), 38

breast cancer, 90
breath shield, 5
bruising, 59, 104, 113
bubbles, under contact lens, 128, 129, 133, 134
bulb and bulb housing, 6-8, 18
bulbar conjunctiva, 36-37, 38
bullae, 46, 72
burn(s), 59, 88-89, 110
burning sensation, 120
BUT (tear break up time), 38
buttonhole, corneal, 108

cancer, 61, 90, 91
Candida albicans infections, 90
canthi, 34
capsule, lens, 44
    opacity of, 80, 116
capsulotomy, 80
carcinoma, 61, 90, 91
carotid artery disease, 90
caruncle, 35
cataract. *See also* Intraocular lens
    complicated, 81
    congenital, 81
    coronary, 81
    cortical, 80-82
    definition of, 80
    formation of, 111, 112
    nuclear sclerotic, 81, 82, 83
    polar, 81
    posterior subscapular, 81, 82
    postoperative, 110, 112, 115, 116
    surgery for, 111, 115-116
    types of, 81
cell(s)
    anterior chamber, 112
        in corneal surgery, 105-106
        grading of, 75-76
        illumination of, 49, 50
        postoperative, 105-106, 112
    corneal epithelium, 105-106. *See also* cornea, infiltrates in
cellulitis, 86
centration
    of contact lens, 125, 126-127, 130
    of intraocular lens, 111
chalazion, 61
chemical burns, 88
chemosis, 63, 104, 111
chickenpox, 90
children
    cataracts in, 81
    pupil size in, 43
    slit lamp examination of, 12, 14-15
chin rest and chin rest papers, 8, 9, 12, 14-15
Chlamydia infections, 90
cilia, 35. *See also* lashes
ciliary flush, 63, 64, 114
ciliary muscle, 43
cleaning
    of contact lenses, 124, 128-130, 132
    of slit lamp equipment, 8-9
closed angle, 75
closure, incomplete, of lids, 104
cobalt blue filter, 5, 20, 38, 131
collarette, 42, 59
coloboma, 59, 77
colon cancer, 90
conformer, for enucleation, 105, 113
congenital cataract, 81

conical (pinpoint) slit beam, 25, 49
conjunctiva. *See also* injection
    appearance of, 36-37
    in contact lens wear, 124, 125
    cyst of, 63
    edema of, 105, 112, 113, 114, 116
    examination of, 21, 23, 26
    findings in, 63-66
    laceration of, 89
conjunctivitis, 86
    giant papillary, 87, 128
contact dermatitis, 86
contact lens evaluation, 6, 123-134
    bandage, 109, 114, 124, 126
    bifocal, 127, 129, 133
    in loose fit, 128, 131, 132
    prefit, 124
    rigid lens, 129-134
    soft lens, 124-129
    in tight fit, 128, 131, 132
cornea
    abrasions of, 67, 72, 104, 105, 111, 113, 129
    appearance of, 38-40, 124
    burns of, 88-89, 110
    clarity of, 39-40
    contact lens wear and, 124
    diameter of, 67
    dry spots on, 72, 104, 113, 114, 132
    dystrophy of, 67, 86, 87
    edema of (haze)
        in contact lens wear, 128, 133
        grading of, 68
        in infections, 104
        postoperative, 106, 109-110, 112, 114, 115, 116
    endothelium of, 39, 40, 50, 111
    epithelium of, 36, 39-40, 109, 112
        postoperative, 105-106, 111
        in refractive surgery, 108
    examination of, 21-22, 26, 38-40
    folds in, 111
    hypoxia of, 128, 133
    illumination techniques for, 46-48, 50, 52
    infections of, 104, 128
    infiltrates in, 68
        in contact lens wear, 133
        postoperative, 107, 109, 114, 115
    inflammation of. *See* keratitis
    layers of, 39-40
    neovascularization of, 71-72
    opacities of, 47, 53, 54, 70, 106, 114
    pannus of, 70
    recurrent erosion of, 88
    vs. sclera, 38
    sclerotic scatter in, 52, 128
    scraping, 6
    staining of, 104
        in contact lens wear, 125, 129, 133, 134
        examination of, 22
        grading of, 72-73
        postoperative, 112, 114, 115, 116
    striae of, 71, 111, 114, 115, 116
    surface of, 48
    surgery on, 105-109, 114
    transplantation of, 105-106, 114
    ulcers of, 71
coronary cataract, 81
cortical cataract, 80-82
coverage, of contact lens, 124, 125
craniofacial syndromes, 90

cross hair reticule, 2
crusting, 60
cyst(s), 61, 77, 78, 108

dacryocystitis, 86
dacryocystorhinostomy, 105
decentration, of contact lens, 126
dellen, 46, 67
    in contact lens wear, 124
    postoperative, 105, 107, 114
dendrites, 72, 74
deposits, on contact lens, 124, 125, 129-130
dermatitis, contact, 86
dermis, appearance of, 34
Descemet's membrane, 39-40, 111
diabetes, 90, 112, 118
diffuse illumination, 46, 47
diffusers, 5, 46
dilation
    lens visualization in, 43-44
    for retroillumination, 54
    for transillumination, 55
dimple veiling, in contact lens wear, 133, 134
direct illumination, 46-50, 56
discharge, 63, 120-121
    in contact lens wear, 128
    postoperative, 104, 105, 113
distichia, 60
documentation, 31. *See also* grading, subjective or the
    specific finding to be documented
Down syndrome, 34, 90
drawings, of corneal pathology, 66
drops, instillation of, 28
drugs
    corneal toxicity of, 106
    ocular findings related to, 92-102
    reactions to, 104
dry eye syndrome, 63, 74, 86, 108
dry spots, corneal, 72, 104, 113, 114, 132
dye
    fluorescein. *See* fluorescein dye
    rose bengal, 37, 38, 40, 74
dystrophy, corneal, 67, 86, 87

ectropion, 60, 86, 104
eczema, 90
edema, 60
    conjunctival, 63, 105, 112, 113, 114, 116
    corneal, 68, 104, 106, 109-110
    lid, 104, 105, 111, 113, 116
emphysema, 90
endocarditis, 90
endophthalmitis, 86, 104
endothelium, corneal, 39, 40, 50, 111
entropion, 60, 86, 104
enucleation, 105, 113
epicanthus, 34
epiphora, 63
episclera
    congestion of, 110
    examination of, 5, 21, 38
    findings in, 63-66
episcleritis, 86-87
epithelium, corneal, 39-40, 112
    postoperative, 105-106, 109, 111
    in refractive surgery, 108
erosion, corneal, 115
erythema, 60
eversion, lid, 28-29
examination, slit lamp. *See* slit lamp examination

examination notes
    in contact lens evaluation, 125, 129
    postoperative, 113-116
examiner position, 19
excimer laser surgery, 107-109
exophthalmos, 87
exposure keratitis, 104
external eye
    appearance of, 37-40
    examination of, 2
    findings of, 59-62
    postoperative examination notes, 113-116
external ocular adnexa, 34-37
extraocular muscles, 105, 113
eye drops, 28, 104
eyebrows, 34
eyelashes. *See* lashes
eyelid(s). *See* lid(s)
eyepieces, 2, 16-17

facial deformity syndromes, 90
filaments, corneal, 68
filter(s), 5
    cobalt blue, 5, 20, 38, 131
    diffuser, 5, 46
    green, 5, 20
    neutral density, 46
    Wrattan, 131
findings, ocular, 58-84. *See also* documentation
    absence of, 58-59
    of anterior chamber and angles, 75-76
    of conjunctiva, 63-66
    in contact lens wear, 123-134
    of cornea, 66-75
    of episclera, 63-66
    external (lid/lacrimal), 59-62
    of globe, 62-84
    in infection, 104
    of intraocular lens, 80-84
    of iris, 77-78
    of lens, 80-84
    measurement in, 59
    medication-related, 92-102
    in ocular diseases, 86-88
    in ocular trauma, 88-89
    postoperative, 105-116
    of pupil, 77-79
    of sclera, 63-66
    subjective grading system for, 58-59
    in systemic diseases and conditions, 89-92
    tears, 62-63
    of vitreous, 84
fixation and fixation light, 5, 8, 18
flap, in LASIK surgery, 108, 114
flare, anterior chamber, 76, 105, 112
Fleisher ring, 5, 68
fluid exchange, 112
fluorescein dye, 40
    in contact lens evaluation, 129, 131, 132
    corneal staining with. *See* cornea, staining of
    filter for, 5
    postoperative, 104, 106, 107
    in tear film evaluation, 38
focusing
    in illumination, 49, 50
    oculars, 17
    slit lamp, 2, 19, 28
folds, corneal, 111
follicles, conjunctival, 63
forehead rest, 9, 17

foreign body sensation, 6, 64, 68, 89, 106, 120
fornix, 36, 37
froth, 60
fundus, retroillumination from (red reflex), 54
fundus contact lens, 6
fuse replacement, 8

gas-permeable (rigid) contact lenses, 129-134
German measles, 90
ghost vessels, 68
giant cell arteritis, 92
giant papillary conjunctivitis, 87, 128
glands, 34-35, 60
glaucoma, 40-41
    open angle, 88
    pigmentary, 88
    surgery for, 109-110
glide plate, 8-9
globe
    examination of, 23
    findings of, 62-84
    perforated, 89
    postoperative examination notes, 113-116
Goldmann tonometer, 6
goniolens, 6, 40
gonorrhea, 90
gout, 86, 90
grading, subjective, 58-59
    angles, 75
    anterior chamber cells, 76
    cataracts, 82, 83
    corneal haze, 68
    corneal staining, 73
    corneal vascularization, 72
    injection, 64
green filter, 5, 20
growths, 120
guttata, corneal, 68

haptics, 11, 44
hay fever, 90
haze, corneal. *See* cornea, edema of
head rest unit, 5, 12-14
head tremors, examination with, 15
headache, 120
hemangioma, 61
hemorrhage, subconjunctival, 65, 105, 106-107, 109-110, 111, 113, 115, 116
herpes simplex virus infections, 87, 90
herpes zoster, 91
high blood pressure, 90
histoplasmosis, 90
history, patient, 117-122
hordeola, 61
horizontal prism light source, 2, 3, 6, 7
Hruby lens, 6, 17
Hudson-Stahli line, 68
human immunodeficiency virus infection, ocular findings in, 89
hygiene, in contact lens wear, 124, 128-130
hyperopia, glaucoma risk in, 41
hypertension, 90
hypervitaminosis, 90
hyphema, 76, 110, 111, 115, 116
hypopyon, 76, 104, 112
hypoxia, corneal, 128, 133

illumination, 45-56
    beam method, 46
    diffuse, 46, 47

direct, 46-50, 56
indirect, 51-56
mnemonic for, 56
pinpoint, 25, 49
proximal, 47, 51
source of, 2-5, 7, 8, 59
specular reflection, 50
tangential, 48
illumination tower, 6
illuminator, 52
indirect illumination, 51-56
indirect retroillumination, 53
infection(s)
    in contact lens wear, 128
    keratitis in, 108
    ocular findings in, 89-92
    postoperative, 104
infectious keratitis, 108
infiltrates, corneal, 68
    in contact lens wear, 133
    postoperative, 107, 109, 114, 115
influenza, 90
injection, 64, 104, 105, 106-107, 109-110, 111, 112, 113, 114, 115, 116
intraocular lens, 82
    anterior chamber, 42
    centration of, 111
    examination of, 23, 44
    findings in, 80-84
    position of, 116
    posterior chamber, 44
intraocular pressure measurement, 6, 40-41
iridectomy, 78, 79
iridodialysis, 77
iridodonesis, 77
iridotomy, laser, 78, 110, 115
iris
    angle blockage by, 41
    atrophy of, 111, 112, 116
    examination of, 23, 27, 42-43
    findings in, 77-80
    intraocular lens fixed to, 42
    retroillumination from, 47, 52-53
    surgery on, 77, 78, 79, 110, 115
    tangential illumination of, 48
    transillumination of, 55, 110
iris rubeosis, 31
iritis, 87
iron lines, 68

jelly bumps, 124
Joseph and Caffrey system, for corneal findings, 66
joystick, 2, 19, 28

Kaposi's sarcoma, 61
keratectomy
    astigmatic, 107
    photorefractive, 107-109
keratitic precipitates, 69-70, 106, 111, 114
keratitis, 87
    in contact lens wear, 129
    infectious, 108
    postoperative, 104, 108, 111, 112, 114, 116
    toxic, 108
keratoconus, 87, 134
keratopathy, 88
    band, 67
    punctate, 72, 75, 106, 108
knobs, for magnification setting, 4, 52
Krukenberg spindles, 70

lacerations, 60, 89
lacrimal system
    findings in, 59-62
    procedures on, 105, 113
LASEK surgery, 107-109
laser surgery, 6
    examination notes for, 114-115
    iridotomy, 78, 110, 115
    refractive, 107-109
    retinal photocoagulation, 112, 116
    trabeculoplasty, 110, 115
lashes
    appearance of, 35
    epilating, 6
    findings in, 60-62
    loss of, 60
    position of, 113
    postoperative problems with, 104
LASIK surgery, 107-109
lateral canthus, 34
leash vessels, conjunctival, 64
lens
    anatomic
        capsule of, 48, 80, 116
        examination of, 2, 23, 27, 43-44
        findings in, 80-84
        opacities of, 80, 110. *See also* cataract
    contact, evaluation. *See* contact lens evaluation
    intraocular. *See* intraocular lens
    slit lamp, 2, 6, 8, 17, 40
        cleaning, 8
        high power indirect, 6
        mirror, 6
leprosy, 90
lesion, 60
leukemia, 91
levator muscle, surgery on, 104
levers, for magnification setting, 4
lid(s)
    blinking of. *See* blink(ing)
    burns of, 89
    closure of, 60, 104
    in contact lens wear, 124
    crusted, 120
    edema of, 104, 105, 111, 113, 116, 121
    eversion of, 28-29
    examination of, 21, 25
    findings in, 59-62, 121
    inflammation of, 86
    laceration of, 89
    lag of, 60
    margin of, 34-35
    notching of, 60
    position of, 37, 60, 113
    retraction of, 60
    surgery on, 104, 113
light source, for slit lamp, 2-5, 19, 20-23
limbal injection (ciliary flush), 64
limbus
    appearance of, 36, 38
    contact lens coverage of, 124, 126
loupe, 37
lung cancer, 91
lupus, 91

magnification, 2, 4, 18-19
    for corneal examination, 39
    dial for, 28
    vs. illumination techniques, 46-55
    for normal eye, 34

for pinpoint illumination, 49
for retroillumination, 54
for specular reflection, 5
suggestion for, 20
for tangential illumination, 48
for transillumination, 554
maintenance, of slit lamp, 6-9
malaria, 91
malnutrition, 91
Marfan's syndrome, 91
matter. *See* discharge
measles, 91
measurement, of findings, 59
medial canthus, 34
medications
    corneal toxicity of, 106
    ocular findings related to, 92-102
    reactions to, 104
    topical, 97-102
meibomian glands, packed, 60
melanoma, 61, 91
menopause, 91
milia, 61
mirror lens, 6, 8
mnemonic, illumination, 56
mole, 61, 78
molluscum contagiosum, 61
mononucleosis, 91
movement, of contact lens, 124, 125, 126, 129, 130
mucin layer, 37-38
multiple sclerosis, 91
mumps, 91
muscle(s)
    extraocular, 105, 113
    iris, 42-43, 105
muscular dystrophy, 91
myasthenia gravis, 91
myopia, 41, 107-109

narrow angles, 75
nasal angle, 22, 41
nasolacrimal obstruction, 88
necrosis, anterior segment, 111
neovascularization, corneal, 71-72, 106, 114, 128
nerve fibers, in cornea, 40
nerve loop, on sclera, 38
neurofibromatosis, 91
neutral density filter, 5, 46
nevus (mole), 61, 78
nuclear sclerosis, of lens, 81, 82, 83
nucleus, of lens, 44, 81, 82, 83
nystagmus, 16

objective findings, 58
objective lens, 2
observation tube, 6
occlusive vascular disease, 91
ocular(s), 28
    adjustment of, 16-17
    power of, 2
ocular adnexa, 2, 34-37
ocular diseases, findings in, 86-88
ocular medications, 97-102
ocular trauma, 88-90
oculomotor nerve palsy, 92
oculoplastic surgery, 104-105, 113
opacities
    capsule, 80, 116
    corneal, 47, 53, 54, 70, 106, 114
    lens, 80, 110

vitreous, 84
open angle glaucoma, 88
optic nerve, 6, 41

pachymeter, 6
pain
    eye, 119
    in glaucoma, 41
    in infection, 104
    postoperative, 111
    slit lamp examination with, 16
palpebral conjunctiva, 36-37, 38
pannus, corneal, 70
papillae, 65
parathyroid disorders, 91
Parkinson's disease, 91
patient education, for examination, 12-16
patient history, implications of, 117-122
peaked pupil, 79
peptic ulcer disease, 91
perforated globe, 89
peripheral iridectomy, 78
phacoemulsification, 111
phlyctenule, 70
photography, 6, 46
photorefractive keratectomy, 107-109
physical symptoms, in history, 119-122
pigmentary glaucoma, 88
pinguecula, 65
pinpoint slit beam, 25, 49
plica semilunaris, 36
polar cataract, 81
port wine stain, 62
positioning
    examiner, 19
    patient, for slit lamp examination, 5-6, 12-16, 28
posterior chamber, 40
    intraocular lens in, 44
posterior segment, 40, 44
posterior subscapular cataract, 81, 82, 83
postoperative examination, 105-116
potential acuity meter, 6
power
    electric
        suggestion for, 20
        turning on, 17-18
    magnification. *See* magnification
precipitates, 69-70, 83, 84, 106, 111, 114
PRK (photorefractive keratectomy), 107-109
prolapse, conjunctival, 113
protocol, for slit lamp examination, 20-27, 29
proximal illumination, 47, 51
pseudoexfoliation, 83, 84
psoriasis, 91
pterygium, 70, 106-107, 114
ptosis, 28, 62, 111, 115
puncta, 6, 35, 62
punctate epithelial erosion, 72, 75
punctate keratopathy, 72, 75, 106, 108
pupil(s)
    examination of, 23, 27, 43
    findings in, 77-80
    intraocular lens fixed to, 42
    postoperative, 110, 111, 112, 115, 116
    reaction of, 43
    size differences in, 120
pupillary distance, 17

radiation burns, 89
rash, 122

recurrent erosion syndrome, 88
recurrent lesions, 113
red reflex, 54, 55
red-free (green) filter, 5, 20
redness, 122, 124
    in contact lens wear, 128
    in glaucoma, 41
    postoperative, 104, 105, 107, 113
reflex, red, 54, 55
reflux, from punctum, 62
refractive surgery, 107-109
rejection, of corneal transplant, 106, 114
retina, surgery on, 111-112, 116
retroillumination, 52-54
    indirect, 53
    iris, 47
rheumatoid arthritis, 91
rigid contact lenses, 129-134
rosacea, 91
rose bengal dye, 37, 38, 40, 74
rubella, 91
rubeola, 91
rubeosis, iris, 79
rust ring, 71

safety, in maintenance, 6, 8
sarcoidosis, 91
scarring, 71, 104, 106, 113, 114
sclera
    examination of, 21, 38
    findings in, 63-66
    inflammation of (scleritis), 88
    structure of, 38-39
scleral buckle, 111, 116
scleritis, 88
scleroderma, 91
sclerotic scatter, 52, 128
seborrheic keratosis, 61
sector iridectomy, 79
Seidel's sign, 106, 114
shingles, 91
sickle cell disease, 91
sinus problems, 92
skin
    appearance of, 34
    rash of, 122
    sloughing of, 113
skin tags, 61
slit beam
    color of, 20-23
    control of, 2, 4
    focusing of, 2, 17, 19, 28
    height of, 20-23, 25, 38
    illumination techniques for, 45-56
    manipulation of, 18, 19
    pinpoint, 25, 49
    vertical, 24
    width of, 2, 9, 17, 20-25, 38, 41
slit lamp examination, 11-31
    of children, 12, 14-15
    documentation of, 29, 31
    fixation in, 18
    focusing in, 2, 17, 19, 28
    light source manipulation in, 19
    magnification in, 2, 4, 18-19
    ocular eyepiece adjustment in, 16-17
    patient education for, 12-16
    positioning for, 5-6, 12-16
    problematic, 85-102
        contact lens, 123-134

medications and, 92-102
    in ocular diseases, 86-88
    in ocular trauma, 88-89
    postoperative, 103-116
    in systemic diseases and conditions, 89-92
    protocol for, 20-27, 29
    special procedures in, 28-29
slit lamp microscope, 1-9
    additional equipment for, 6
    examination with. *See* slit lamp examination
    focusing of, 2, 17, 19, 28
    illumination in, 2, 3, 7, 8, 19, 59
    instrumentation for, 2-6
    light source for, 2-5, 7, 8, 19, 59
    magnification settings for, 2, 4, 18-19, 46-55
    maintenance of, 6-9
    powering up, 17-18
    therapeutic use of, 6
    troubleshooting for, 18, 28
smallpox, 92
smoking, 92
socket, after enucleation, 105, 113
soft contact lenses, 124-129
specular reflection, 50
squamous cell carcinoma, 61
stage, position of, 2, 12, 19-23, 29
staining, corneal, 104, 112, 115
    in contact lens wear, 125, 129, 133
    dyes for. *See* fluorescein dye; rose bengal dye
    examination of, 22
    grading of, 72-73
    postoperative, 114, 116
strabismus, 16
strands
    iris, 78
    vitreous, 84
striae, corneal, 71, 111, 114, 115, 116, 128
stroma, 40, 105, 107, 108, 109, 111
subconjunctival hemorrhage, 65, 105, 106-107, 109-110, 111, 113, 115, 116
subjective grading system. *See* grading, subjective
subluxation, of lens, 83
superficial punctate keratopathy, 72, 74
superior fornix, 37
surgery
    cataract, 111, 115-116
    corneal, 105-109, 114
    glaucoma, 109-110
    iris, 77, 78, 79, 110, 115
    laser. *See* laser surgery
    levator muscle, 104
    oculoplastic, 104-105, 113
    postoperative examination in, 105-116
    refractive, 107-109
    retinal, 111-112, 116
sutures
    broken, 104, 105, 111, 113, 114, 115
    trimming, 6
swelling. *See* edema
sympathetic ophthalmia, 104
symptoms
    physical, 119-122
    visual, 118-119
synechiae, 79, 80, 110, 111, 112, 115, 116
syneresis scintillans, 84
systemic diseases and conditions, ocular findings in, 89-92

tangential illumination, 48
tear break up time, 38

tear film
    abnormal, 122
    composition of, 37
    in corneal transplant, 106
    evaluation in contact lens wear, 124, 129, 132
    examination of, 21
    findings in, 62-63
    normal, 37-38
    postoperative, 104, 105, 113
tear gland, prolapsed, 65
temporal arteritis, 92
test rod, focusing, 17
thermal burns, 89
third nerve palsy, 92
thyroid disease, 92
tight contact lens, 128
tonometer, 6, 12, 40-41, 109-110
Topcon slit lamp, 3
topical medications, 97-102
toxic cataract, 81
toxic keratitis, 108
toxoplasmosis, 92
trabeculoplasty, 110, 115
transformer, 2, 18
transillumination, iris, 55, 110, 112
transplantation, corneal, 105-106
trauma, ocular, findings in, 88-89
tremors, examination with, 15
trichiasis, 62, 104
troubleshooting, 18
truncation, of contact lens, 127
tuberculosis, 92
Tyndall's phenomenon, 49

ulcer(s), corneal, 71
ultrasound, 6

ultraviolet burns, 89
uveitis, 88

vaccinia infections, 92
vacuoles, lens, 84
varicella, 92
variola, 92
vascularization. *See* blood vessels; neovascularization
vertical illumination light source, 2, 3, 7, 8, 59
video camera, 6
visual symptoms, in history, 118-119
vitamin deficiencies, 92
vitrectomy, 112, 116
vitreous
    in anterior chamber, 76, 116
    anterior face of, 44
    examination of, 2, 23
    findings in, 84
    opacities of, 84
voltage, 2, 18
von Recklinghausen's disease, 91

Waring and Laibson scheme, for corneal pathology, 66
warts, 61
wheelchair, slit lamp examination with, 15
wound gape, 113, 114, 115
Wrattan filter, 131
wrinkles, corneal, 108

xanthelasma, 61

Y-sutures, 44

zonular cataract, 81
zonules, 43-44

Build Your Library

Along with this title, we publish numerous products on a variety of topics. We are sure that you will find the below titles to be an essential addition to your library. Order your copies today or contact us for a copy of our latest catalog for additional product information.

CERTIFIED OPHTHALMIC ASSISTANT EXAM REVIEW MANUAL, SECOND EDITION

Janice K. Ledford, COMT

192 pp., Soft Cover, 2003, ISBN 1-55642-642-9, Order #66429, **$36.95**

The *Certified Ophthalmic Assistant Exam Review Manual, Second Edition* is an essential resource for anyone preparing to become certified as an ophthalmic assistant. With over 650 exam-style questions and explanatory answers, illustrations, and photographs, this user-friendly text is excellent for both learning and reviewing important eye care topics.

THE LITTLE EYE BOOK: A PUPIL'S GUIDE TO UNDERSTANDING OPHTHALMOLOGY

Janice K. Ledford, COMT and Roberto Pineda II, MD

160 pp., Soft Cover, 2002, ISBN 1-55642-560-0, Order #65600, **$18.95**

The Little Eye Book: A Pupil's Guide to Understanding Ophthalmology is an easy-to-understand introduction to the field of eye care. This book is written with the non-physician in mind, so you won't be bogged down with heavy details, yet every basic fact that you need is right here.

HANDBOOK OF CLINICAL OPHTHALMOLOGY FOR EYECARE PROFESSIONALS

Janice K. Ledford, COMT

384 pp., Soft Cover, 2002, ISBN 1-55642-464-7, Order #64647, **$36.95**

This book serves as an ophthalmic pocket companion for the eyecare paraprofessional. With 100 tables and illustrations throughout the text, the reader will find this an extremely useful guide covering essentially every aspect of patient care.

Contact Us

SLACK Incorporated, Professional Book Division
6900 Grove Road, Thorofare, NJ 08086
1-800-257-8290/1-856-848-1000, Fax: 1-856-853-5991
orders@slackinc.com or www.slackbooks.com

ORDER FORM

QUANTITY	TITLE	ORDER #	PRICE
	COA® Exam Review Manual, Second Edition	66429	$36.95
	The Little Eye Book	65600	$18.95
	Handbook of Clinical Ophthalmology for Eyecare Professionals	64647	$36.95
		Subtotal	$
		Applicable state and local tax will be added to your purchase	$
		Handling	$5.00
		Total	$

Name: _____

Address: _____

City: _____ State: _____ Zip: _____

Phone: _____ Fax: _____

Email: _____

- Check enclosed (Payable to SLACK Incorporated)_____

- Charge my: ____ [AMEX] ____ [VISA] ____ [MasterCard]

Account #: _____

Exp. date: _____ Signature: _____

Security Code _____

NOTE: *Prices are subject to change without notice.*
Shipping charges will apply.
Shipping and handling charges are non-returnable.

CODE: 328